Practical Guide to Hereditary Breast and Ovarian Cancer IV

Masami Arai • Shinji Ohno • Masayuki Sekine
Editors

Practical Guide to Hereditary Breast and Ovarian Cancer IV

Annual Meeting of the Japanese Organization of Hereditary Breast and Ovarian Cancer 2024

Springer

Editors
Masami Arai
Department of Clinical Genetics
Graduate School of Medicine
Juntendo University
Bunkyo-ku, Tokyo, Japan

Shinji Ohno
Department of Breast-Thyroid Surgery
Sagara Hospital
Kagoshima, Japan

Masayuki Sekine
Department of Obstetrics and Gynecology
Graduate School of Medical Science
University of the Ryukyus
Ginowan, Okinawa, Japan

ISBN 978-981-95-6579-5   ISBN 978-981-95-6580-1 (eBook)
https://doi.org/10.1007/978-981-95-6580-1

This Springer imprint is published by the registered company Springer Nature Singapore Pte Ltd.
The registered company address is: 152 Beach Road, #21-01/04 Gateway East, Singapore 189721, Singapore

Foreword

This Year Book compiles the outcomes of the 4th Annual Meeting of the Japanese Organization of Hereditary Breast and Ovarian Cancer (JOHBOC) held in 2024. This meeting provided a valuable opportunity to share advances in research and clinical practice, focusing on hereditary breast and ovarian cancer (HBOC), and to discuss the future direction of care.

The symposium sessions covered a wide range of important and practical topics. These included the latest insights into the evaluation of homologous recombination deficiency (HRD) in gynecology, medical care for unaffected BRCA pathogenic variant carriers in breast oncology, the integration of new findings into HBOC clinical practice in genetics, challenges in reproductive medicine and preimplantation genetic testing for monogenic diseases (PGT-M) in obstetrics and gynecology, as well as cutting-edge research on carcinogenic mechanisms and therapeutic strategies in HBOC from a basic science perspective.

In addition, this Annual Meeting emphasized the importance of incorporating the voices and perspectives of patients and their families into clinical practice and research. HBOC management is not limited to physicians and researchers, but requires the collaboration of patients, families, genetic counselors, nurses, psychologists, as well as communities and policymakers. Patient-centered discussions highlighted the need to create a healthcare system where medical decision-making based on genetic information is supported not only in the clinic but also at the societal level. Such efforts will promote personalized medicine in daily practice and contribute to greater public understanding and the development of supportive healthcare policies.

I would like to express my sincere gratitude to Drs. Masami Arai, Shinji Ohno, and Masayuki Sekine for their significant contributions to the editing of this book. I hope that this Year Book will serve not only as a source of knowledge for healthcare professionals involved in HBOC and related cancers but also as a foundation for building a comprehensive, patient- and family-centered healthcare system in society.

Finally, I would like to express my deepest condolences for the late Dr. Seigo Nakamura, a world-renowned pioneer who led this field for many years and made tremendous efforts for the benefit of numerous patients through this Year Book.

Tokyo, Japan
August 2025

Nao Suzuki

Editorial Board

Contents

Advances in Assisted Reproductive Technology and PGT-M

Excellent General Presentation

JOHBOC Registration

Advances in Basic Science

DNA Damage Response and Immune Checkpoint: Recent Advances in Basic Science

Naoe Taira Nihira

Abstract The breast and ovarian cancer susceptibility genes BRCA1 and BRCA2 are essential for preserving genomic stability, primarily through their role in homologous recombination (HR) repair of DNA double-strand breaks. Consequently, cells harboring germline or somatic mutations in BRCA1 or BRCA2 lack DNA repair via HR and are predisposed to carcinogenesis. Poly (ADP-ribose) polymerase (PARP) inhibitors represent a therapeutic strategy that exploits synthetic lethality in HR-deficient cells. However, PARP inhibition also activates the cyclic GMP-AMP synthase (cGAS)-stimulator of interferon genes (STING) pathway, a key regulator of inflammation, and induces expression of the immune checkpoint molecule programmed death-ligand 1 (PD-L1). These effects suggest that immune checkpoint inhibitors (ICIs) may be particularly effective in combination with PARP inhibitors for HR-deficient cancers by counteracting PD-L1-mediated immune evasion. This review examines the molecular mechanisms through which genotoxic stress drives inflammation in HR-deficient cancers and discusses emerging strategies to improve ICI-based immunotherapy by targeting inflammation-associated pathways.

Keywords DNA damage · Inflammation · PARP inhibitor · PD-L1 · cGAS-STING

1 Introduction

Hereditary breast and ovarian cancer syndrome is a well-established inherited cancer predisposition primarily linked to germline mutations in the BRCA1 and BRCA2 genes. Females with BRCA1 mutations have an estimated lifetime risk of breast cancer of about 60% and ovarian cancer of 40–50%. For BRCA2 mutation

N. T. Nihira (✉)
Department of Translational Oncology, St. Marianna University Graduate School of Medicine, Kawasaki, Japan
e-mail: nnihira@marianna-u.ac.jp

M. Arai et al. (eds.), *Practical Guide to Hereditary Breast and Ovarian Cancer IV*,
https://doi.org/10.1007/978-981-95-6580-1_1

carriers, the respective risks are 40% for breast cancer and 10–20% for ovarian cancer [2, 14, 42]. The development of molecularly targeted agents, such as poly (ADP-ribose) polymerase (PARP) inhibitors, has significantly advanced treatment options for patients with BRCA1/2 mutations [5, 13]. However, PARP inhibition also activates the cyclic GMP-AMP synthase (cGAS)-stimulator of interferon genes (STING) pathway, a critical regulator of inflammatory signaling, while simultaneously inducing expression of the immune checkpoint protein programmed death-ligand 1 (PD-L1). Immune checkpoint inhibitors (ICIs) have therefore gained attention, as BRCA1/2 deficiency is associated with increased PD-L1/programmed death-1 (PD-1) expression, underscoring the immunologic consequences of homologous recombination (HR) deficiency [45]. This review explores therapeutic strategies for patients with BRCA1/2 mutations, emphasizing molecular mechanisms and their implications for targeted and immunotherapeutic interventions.

2 Genomic Instability as a Therapeutic Vulnerability

DNA repair mechanisms activated in response to DNA damage depend on the cell cycle phases [17]. DNA lesions arising during the G1 phase are mainly repaired through non-homologous end joining (NHEJ), a pathway that often produces small insertions or deletions [21]. In contrast, damage during the S and G2 phases is primarily repaired by HR, a high-fidelity mechanism. Because BRCA1 and BRCA2 are essential for HR, germline or somatic mutations in either gene disrupt HR function [41]. In the absence of HR, cells rely on error-prone repair pathways such as alternative end joining (Alt-EJ), which promote genomic instability and malignant transformation [6, 10]. Consequently, HR deficiency caused by BRCA1/2 mutations increases the risk of breast and ovarian cancers. PARP is a key enzyme in Alt-EJ repair. Pharmacologic inhibition of PARP selectively targets HR-deficient cells, a therapeutic approach termed synthetic lethality. In this model, simultaneous impairment of BRCA1/2- and PARP1-mediated repair causes cell death, whereas disruption of either pathway alone is non-lethal. This concept underlies the clinical efficacy of PARP inhibitors in HR-deficient tumors [5, 13]. When DNA lesions accumulate in HR-proficient cells exposed to PARP inhibition, a DNA damage response is initiated, and the cell attempts to transiently arrest the cell cycle. Detection of double-strand breaks (DSBs) activates the G2/M checkpoint, promoting temporary arrest. However, in HR-deficient cells lacking BRCA1 or BRCA2, repair is ineffective, leading to unresolved damage. Checkpoint control subsequently fails, and cells enter mitosis with unrepaired DNA. This aberrant mitotic entry produces mitotic catastrophe, characterized by chromosomal mis-segregation, breaks, and spindle apparatus defects [34, 39]. These abnormalities prevent accurate cell division and trigger lethal stress. In addition, persistent DNA damage and cycle dysregulation increase mitochondrial membrane permeability, releasing pro-apoptotic factors such as cytochrome c into the cytosol. This event activates the intrinsic apoptotic pathway and drives programmed cell death.

3 Genomic Instability and the Inflammatory Tumor Microenvironment

Accumulating evidence indicates that genomic instability is closely associated with upregulation of PD-L1 in cancer cells. Sato et al. identified BRCA2 and Ku70/80 as key regulators in an siRNA screen targeting DSB repair genes. Depletion of these molecules enhanced PD-L1 expression after X-ray irradiation or PARP inhibition [36]. Mechanistically, treatment of HR-deficient cells with PARP inhibitors activates the cGAS-STING pathway, inducing inflammation and elevating expression of the immune checkpoint molecule PD-L1 [19]. DNA damage-induced upregulation is primarily linked to inflammation-related mechanisms mediated by the cGAS-STING pathway [9, 11, 40] or the STAT1/3-IRF1 signaling axis [36].

3.1 cGAS-STING Pathway

The cGAS-STING pathway is a cytosolic DNA-sensing mechanism, typically activated by infection with pathogens or DNA viruses, and is essential for innate immunity. Cellular double-stranded DNA (dsDNA) generated by DNA damage or oncogene-induced replication stress accumulates in micronuclei, where it activates the cGAS-STING pathway and innate immunity [28]. The double-stranded DNA (dsDNA) within micronuclei is released into the cytoplasm through phosphorylation of the nuclear envelope (NE) component Lamin A/C by ATR and CDK1 [20, 23]. Nucleic acids produced by DNA damage are primarily recognized by cGAS. To prevent aberrant activation of the cGAS-STING pathway, cGAS is sequestered by nucleosomes through specific binding to the acidic patch (AP) of histones H2A and H2B. The MRE11-RAD50-NBS1 (MRN) complex promotes release of cGAS from this high-affinity interaction, enabling its mobilization and response to cytosolic dsDNA [8]. Displacement enables cGAS to engage dsDNA and become enzymatically active, catalyzing the production of cyclic GMP-AMP (cGAMP), a secondary messenger. cGAMP binds to STING on the endoplasmic reticulum membrane, triggering conformational activation and translocation to the Golgi apparatus [31]. At the Golgi, STING serves as a signaling hub, recruiting and activating TANK-binding kinase 1 (TBK1) and IκB kinase (IKK) complexes. TBK1 phosphorylates interferon regulatory factor 3 (IRF3), promoting nuclear translocation and induction of type I interferons. In parallel, the IKK complex phosphorylates IκBα, leading to its degradation and nuclear translocation of NF-κB (p65/p50), which drives transcription of pro-inflammatory cytokines including TNF-α, IL-6, and IL-1β (Fig. 1) [1, 4]. Coordinated activation of IRF3 and NF-κB pathways elicits potent antiviral and inflammatory responses, contributing to host defense, tumor immunogenicity, and, under certain conditions, chronic inflammation and autoimmunity. Activation of the cGAS–STING pathway also stimulates antitumor immunity by inducing inflammation. Both downstream transcription factors of cGAS-STING signaling, NF-κB and

IRF3, promote PD-L1 transcription. NF-κB binds directly to the PD-L1 promoter, whereas IRF3 induces type I interferon production, which subsequently upregulates PD-L1 via the STAT or IRF signaling cascade.

3.2 *STAT/IRF Signaling*

As described above, activation of IRF3 through the cGAS-STING pathway promotes transcription of type I interferons, including IFN-α and IFN-β. Both type I and type II interferons are established upstream regulators of PD-L1 expression [16, 29]. The binding of IFN-γ to its receptors IFNGR1 and IFNGR2 activates the JAK2-STAT1 cascade. Phosphorylated STAT1 translocates to the nucleus, inducing transcription of IRF1, a transcription factor that directly binds to the PD-L1 promoter [24, 30]. Sato et al. also demonstrated that ATR and CHK1 activation after radiation-induced DNA damage promotes PD-L1 expression via IRF1 through STAT1/3 [36]. DSB-inducing agents activate the canonical JAK/STAT pathway, where JAK2 activation leads to STAT1 phosphorylation and nuclear translocation. Nuclear STAT1 induces IRF1 transcription, which binds to the PD-L1 promoter and enhances expression [16]. Several chemotherapeutic agents, including 5-fluorouracil (5-FU), gemcitabine, and paclitaxel, increase PD-L1 transcription through STAT1 activation in a JAK2-dependent manner [12]. Camptothecin or etoposide administration

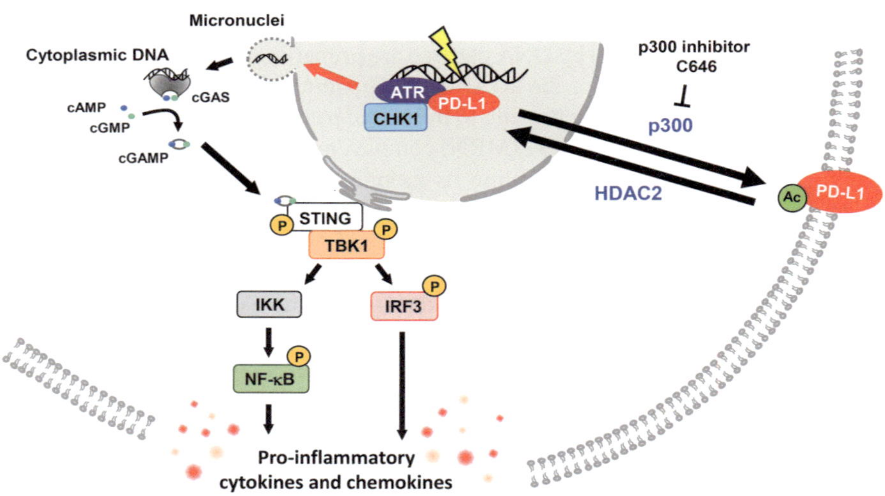

Fig. 1 Schematic diagram of the cGAS-STING pathway. Cytoplasmic DNA generated by genotoxic stress, including chemical agents or UV irradiation, is released from micronuclei and detected by the innate immune sensor cGAS. Upon DNA recognition, cGAS synthesizes the second messenger cGAMP, which activates STING and promotes its translocation from the endoplasmic reticulum to the Golgi apparatus. Activated STING then recruits and activates TBK1, resulting in phosphorylation of IRF3 and NF-κB and induction of pro-inflammatory cytokines and chemokines

similarly induces STAT1/3 phosphorylation and IRF1 expression [36]. Furthermore, the PARP inhibitor Olaparib stimulates STAT1/3 phosphorylation, and these heterodimers directly bind to the PD-L1 promoter [35].

4 Implications of DNA Damage-Induced PD-L1 Expression

PD-L1 is a key immune checkpoint molecule that maintains immune tolerance. Under physiological conditions, PD-L1 is expressed on antigen-presenting cells and certain non-immune cells including cancer cells, where it binds to PD-1 on activated T cells. This interaction delivers inhibitory signals that suppress T cell proliferation, cytokine production, and cytotoxicity, thereby preventing excessive immune responses and autoimmunity. In the tumor microenvironment, many cancer cells exploit this pathway by upregulating PD-L1 in response to IFN signals. This immune evasion mechanism enables tumor cells to suppress antitumor T cell activity, fostering immune tolerance toward malignant cells. ICIs, including anti-PD-1 and anti-PD-L1 antibodies, block the PD-1/PD-L1 interaction and restore T cell function. By releasing this inhibitory brake, ICIs reactivate tumor-specific T cells, enhance cytokine production, and promote immune-mediated tumor cell killing.

Tumors are often categorized as "cold," with few infiltrating $CD8^+$ T cells, or "hot," enriched with $CD8^+$ T cells. ICIs demonstrate greater efficacy in hot tumors, where PD-L1 expression is typically high. Abundant tumor-infiltrating lymphocytes (TILs) correlate with favorable outcomes after PD-1/PD-L1 blockade, underscoring the link between PD-L1 expression and inflammation [18, 27]. Although predominantly localized on the cell surface, PD-L1 is also present in the nucleus [15]. Unlike its membrane-associated role in immune evasion, nuclear PD-L1 regulates transcription of inflammation- and immunity-related genes. Mechanistically, nuclear PD-L1 acts as a DNA damage sensor in coordination with ATR and activates downstream CHK1 [22, 32]. PD-L1 also cooperates with ATR to amplify cGAS-STING pathway activation. While PD-L1 is a downstream target of cGAS-STING, nuclear PD-L1 can, in turn, promote cGAS-STING activation, establishing a positive feedback loop. In a mouse model engineered to express nuclear-localized PD-L1 (nPD-L1) through substitution of Lys249 and Lys251 with alanine, tumors exhibited increased TILs and heightened inflammatory responses [26]. These findings suggest that nuclear PD-L1 strengthens inflammatory signaling and reshapes the tumor immune microenvironment into a "hot" state.

5 Expanding Inflammation as a Strategy for ICI Combination Therapy

5.1 STING Agonist

STING agonists activate the innate immune STING pathway, inducing type I IFNs and pro-inflammatory cytokines through the TBK1-IRF3 axis. This promotes dendritic cell maturation and T cell priming, thereby enhancing antitumor immunity. In 2020, two small-molecule compounds, MSA-2 and SR-717, were identified as novel STING agonists. These agents stabilize the active conformation of STING and promote the transcription of inflammatory cytokines, thereby leading to the activation of dendritic cells and subsequent stimulation of $CD8^+$ T cell responses in mice [7, 33]. In humans, STING activation within the tumor microenvironment may likewise elicit antitumor responses and tumor regression, particularly in immunologically "cold" tumors with limited T cell infiltration. STING agonists may also act synergistically with ICIs, chemotherapy, or radiation, suggesting their potential utility in combination therapy. Several STING agonists, including ADU-S100, MK-1454, and BMS-986301, are currently under clinical evaluation. Most of these agents are cyclic dinucleotide analogs or non-nucleotide small molecules administered intratumorally or systemically. Early-phase trials are investigating their safety, tolerability, and preliminary efficacy, either as monotherapy or in combination with ICIs. Beyond small molecules, lipid nanoparticles (LNPs) have emerged as carriers for cancer vaccines, though peptide or mRNA vaccines often elicit modest T cell responses. Zhou et al. developed an LNP platform co-delivering tumor antigens with Svg3, a cGAS agonist, to enhance type I interferon responses. This strategy improved antigen presentation and antigen-specific $CD8^+$ T cell activation in lymph nodes. In preclinical models, Svg3-loaded LNP vaccines combined with ICI enhanced antitumor immunity and therapeutic efficacy [46]. However, chronic or excessive STING activation may promote metastasis and immunosuppressive remodeling of the tumor microenvironment [3]. These findings highlight the importance of careful dosing, scheduling, and patient selection in clinical applications.

5.2 p300 Inhibitor C646

Nuclear translocation of PD-L1 is promoted by deacetylation of lysine residues within its cytoplasmic domain by HDAC2 [15, 44]. Conversely, acetylation by the acetyltransferase p300 facilitates PD-L1 localization to the plasma membrane [32]. C646, a selective p300 inhibitor, increases nuclear translocation of PD-L1 (Fig. 1). As described above, nuclear PD-L1 enhances the activation of the cGAS-STING cascade; therefore, treatment with C646 further increases the transcription of pro-inflammatory cytokines following DNA damage-induced cGAS-STING activation [32]. This effect was absent in PD-L1 knockout cells, suggesting that C646 acts selectively on PD-L1-positive cells and may serve as a candidate for combination therapy with ICIs.

6 Perspectives

In tumors characterized by genomic instability, including those with HR deficiency, impaired DNA repair mechanisms drive tumor development. The resulting mutation accumulation produces aberrant proteins that act as neoantigens, recognized by immune cells to trigger antitumor and inflammatory responses. Cytokines such as IFNs, produced during this response, stimulate antitumor immunity but also induce PD-L1 transcription, thereby influencing the efficacy of ICIs. Beyond this neoantigen-driven mechanism, DNA damage in HR-deficient cells can directly induce PD-L1 transcription via the cGAS-STING pathway, independent of infection-related inflammation. Genomic instability thus heightens susceptibility to inflammatory signaling, promoting PD-L1 upregulation and immune tolerance.

In triple-negative breast cancer (TNBC) with genomic instability, PD-L1 expression is frequently elevated and correlates with clinical benefit from ICI therapy [37, 38]. The therapeutic effect of ICIs in TNBC depends on the tumor immune microenvironment, which can be classified as non-immunoreactive cold tumors or hot tumors enriched with immune cell infiltration [43]. From an immunological perspective, PD-L1-positive cold tumors rarely respond to ICIs, whereas PD-L1-positive hot tumors, despite poor prognosis, demonstrate clinical benefit. Accordingly, combining ICIs with therapies that stimulate inflammatory and immune responses represents a promising strategy to improve ICI efficacy.

It should be noted, however, that chronic activation of the cGAS-STING pathway can promote metastasis by establishing a tumor microenvironment that is simultaneously pro-inflammatory and immunosuppressive. This process involves secretion of pro-metastatic factors such as CCL5 and matrix metalloproteinases (MMPs), as well as STING activation in stromal cells, including cancer-associated fibroblasts and endothelial cells, which facilitates tumor invasion and angiogenesis [3]. Therefore, in inflammation-inducing therapies, concurrent administration of ICIs is essential to prevent immune escape at both primary and metastatic sites.

Inflammation-driven remodeling of the tumor microenvironment may also recruit immunosuppressive populations, including regulatory T cells (Tregs), tumor-associated macrophages (TAMs), and myeloid-derived suppressor cells (MDSCs) [25]. Strategies targeting these cells, such as CTLA-4 antibodies that deplete Tregs, may therefore represent valuable components of inflammation-based cancer immunotherapy. Nevertheless, the mechanisms by which inflammation, particularly cGAS-STING activation, regulates immune cell recruitment and function remain incompletely understood. Further investigation into the inflammatory tumor microenvironment is likely to refine and expand the scope of cancer immunotherapy.

References

1. Abe T, Barber GN. Cytosolic-DNA-mediated, STING-dependent proinflammatory gene induction necessitates canonical NF-kappaB activation through TBK1. J Virol. 2014;88(10):5328–41. https://doi.org/10.1128/JVI.00037-14.
2. Antoniou A, Pharoah PD, Narod S, Risch HA, Eyfjord JE, Hopper JL, Loman N, Olsson H, Johannsson O, Borg A, Pasini B, Radice P, Manoukian S, Eccles DM, Tang N, Olah E, Anton-Culver H, Warner E, Lubinski J, Gronwald J, Gorski B, Tulinius H, Thorlacius S, Eerola H, Nevanlinna H, Syrjakoski K, Kallioniemi OP, Thompson D, Evans C, Peto J, Lalloo F, Evans DG, Easton DF. Average risks of breast and ovarian cancer associated with BRCA1 or BRCA2 mutations detected in case series unselected for family history: a combined analysis of 22 studies. Am J Hum Genet. 2003;72(5):1117–30. https://doi.org/10.1086/375033.
3. Bakhoum SF, Ngo B, Laughney AM, Cavallo JA, Murphy CJ, Ly P, Shah P, Sriram RK, Watkins TBK, Taunk NK, Duran M, Pauli C, Shaw C, Chadalavada K, Rajasekhar VK, Genovese G, Venkatesan S, Birkbak NJ, McGranahan N, Lundquist M, LaPlant Q, Healey JH, Elemento O, Chung CH, Lee NY, Imielenski M, Nanjangud G, Pe'er D, Cleveland DW, Powell SN, Lammerding J, Swanton C, Cantley LC. Chromosomal instability drives metastasis through a cytosolic DNA response. Nature. 2018;553(7689):467–72. https://doi.org/10.1038/nature25432.
4. Balka KR, Louis C, Saunders TL, Smith AM, Calleja DJ, D'Silva DB, Moghaddas F, Tailler M, Lawlor KE, Zhan Y, Burns CJ, Wicks IP, Miner JJ, Kile BT, Masters SL, De Nardo D. TBK1 and IKKepsilon act redundantly to mediate STING-induced NF-kappaB responses in myeloid cells. Cell Rep. 2020;31(1):107492. https://doi.org/10.1016/j.celrep.2020.03.056.
5. Bryant HE, Schultz N, Thomas HD, Parker KM, Flower D, Lopez E, Kyle S, Meuth M, Curtin NJ, Helleday T. Specific killing of BRCA2-deficient tumours with inhibitors of poly(ADP-ribose) polymerase. Nature. 2005;434(7035):913–7. https://doi.org/10.1038/nature03443.
6. Ceccaldi R, Rondinelli B, D'Andrea AD. Repair pathway choices and consequences at the double-Strand break. Trends Cell Biol. 2016;26(1):52–64. https://doi.org/10.1016/j.tcb.2015.07.009.
7. Chin EN, Yu C, Vartabedian VF, Jia Y, Kumar M, Gamo AM, Vernier W, Ali SH, Kissai M, Lazar DC, Nguyen N, Pereira LE, Benish B, Woods AK, Joseph SB, Chu A, Johnson KA, Sander PN, Martinez-Pena F, Hampton EN, Young TS, Wolan DW, Chatterjee AK, Schultz PG, Petrassi HM, Teijaro JR, Lairson LL. Antitumor activity of a systemic STING-activating non-nucleotide cGAMP mimetic. Science. 2020;369(6506):993–9. https://doi.org/10.1126/science.abb4255.
8. Cho MG, Kumar RJ, Lin CC, Boyer JA, Shahir JA, Fagan-Solis K, Simpson DA, Fan C, Foster CE, Goddard AM, Lerner LM, Ellington SW, Wang Q, Wang Y, Ho AY, Liu P, Perou CM, Zhang Q, McGinty RK, Purvis JE, Gupta GP. MRE11 liberates cGAS from nucleosome sequestration during tumorigenesis. Nature. 2024;625(7995):585–92. https://doi.org/10.1038/s41586-023-06889-6.
9. Chopra N, Tovey H, Pearson A, Cutts R, Toms C, Proszek P, Hubank M, Dowsett M, Dodson A, Daley F, Kriplani D, Gevensleben H, Davies HR, Degasperi A, Roylance R, Chan S, Tutt A, Skene A, Evans A, Bliss JM, Nik-Zainal S, Turner NC. Homologous recombination DNA repair deficiency and PARP inhibition activity in primary triple negative breast cancer. Nat Commun. 2020;11(1):2662. https://doi.org/10.1038/s41467-020-16142-7.
10. Ciccia A, Elledge SJ. The DNA damage response: making it safe to play with knives. Mol Cell. 2010, Oct 22;40(2):179–204. https://doi.org/10.1016/j.molcel.2010.09.019.
11. Ding L, Kim HJ, Wang Q, Kearns M, Jiang T, Ohlson CE, Li BB, Xie S, Liu JF, Stover EH, Howitt BE, Bronson RT, Lazo S, Roberts TM, Freeman GJ, Konstantinopoulos PA, Matulonis UA, Zhao JJ. PARP inhibition elicits STING-dependent antitumor immunity in Brca1-deficient ovarian cancer. Cell Rep. 2018;25(11):2972–80 e2975. https://doi.org/10.1016/j.celrep.2018.11.054.

12. Doi T, Ishikawa T, Okayama T, Oka K, Mizushima K, Yasuda T, Sakamoto N, Katada K, Kamada K, Uchiyama K, Handa O, Takagi T, Naito Y, Itoh Y. The JAK/STAT pathway is involved in the upregulation of PD-L1 expression in pancreatic cancer cell lines. Oncol Rep. 2017;37(3):1545–54. https://doi.org/10.3892/or.2017.5399.
13. Farmer H, McCabe N, Lord CJ, Tutt AN, Johnson DA, Richardson TB, Santarosa M, Dillon KJ, Hickson I, Knights C, Martin NM, Jackson SP, Smith GC, Ashworth A. Targeting the DNA repair defect in BRCA mutant cells as a therapeutic strategy. Nature. 2005;434(7035):917–21. https://doi.org/10.1038/nature03445.
14. Ford D, Easton DF, Stratton M, Narod S, Goldgar D, Devilee P, Bishop DT, Weber B, Lenoir G, Chang-Claude J, Sobol H, Teare MD, Struewing J, Arason A, Scherneck S, Peto J, Rebbeck TR, Tonin P, Neuhausen S, Barkardottir R, Eyfjord J, Lynch H, Ponder BA, Gayther SA, Zelada-Hedman M, et al. Genetic heterogeneity and penetrance analysis of the BRCA1 and BRCA2 genes in breast cancer families. The Breast Cancer Linkage Consortium. Am J Hum Genet. 1998;62(3):676–89. https://doi.org/10.1086/301749.
15. Gao Y, Nihira NT, Bu X, Chu C, Zhang J, Kolodziejczyk A, Fan Y, Chan NT, Ma L, Liu J, Wang D, Dai X, Liu H, Ono M, Nakanishi A, Inuzuka H, North BJ, Huang YH, Sharma S, Geng Y, Xu W, Liu XS, Li L, Miki Y, Sicinski P, Freeman GJ, Wei W. Acetylation-dependent regulation of PD-L1 nuclear translocation dictates the efficacy of anti-PD-1 immunotherapy. Nat Cell Biol. 2020;22(9):1064–75. https://doi.org/10.1038/s41556-020-0562-4.
16. Garcia-Diaz A, Shin DS, Moreno BH, Saco J, Escuin-Ordinas H, Rodriguez GA, Zaretsky JM, Sun L, Hugo W, Wang X, Parisi G, Saus CP, Torrejon DY, Graeber TG, Comin-Anduix B, Hu-Lieskovan S, Damoiseaux R, Lo RS, Ribas A. Interferon receptor signaling pathways regulating PD-L1 and PD-L2 expression. Cell Rep. 2019;29(11):3766. https://doi.org/10.1016/j.celrep.2019.11.113.
17. Her J, Bunting SF. How cells ensure correct repair of DNA double-strand breaks. J Biol Chem. 2018, Jul 6;293(27):10502–11. https://doi.org/10.1074/jbc.TM118.000371.
18. Ilie M, Falk AT, Butori C, Chamorey E, Bonnetaud C, Long E, Lassalle S, Zahaf K, Venissac N, Mouroux J, Cohen C, Brambilla E, Marquette CH, Hofman V, Hofman P. PD-L1 expression in basaloid squamous cell lung carcinoma: relationship to PD-1(+) and CD8(+) tumor-infiltrating T cells and outcome. Mod Pathol. 2016;29(12):1552–64. https://doi.org/10.1038/modpathol.2016.149.
19. Jiao S, Xia W, Yamaguchi H, Wei Y, Chen MK, Hsu JM, Hsu JL, Yu WH, Du Y, Lee HH, Li CW, Chou CK, Lim SO, Chang SS, Litton J, Arun B, Hortobagyi GN, Hung MC. PARP inhibitor upregulates PD-L1 expression and enhances cancer-associated immunosuppression. Clin Cancer Res. 2017;23(14):3711–20. https://doi.org/10.1158/1078-0432.CCR-16-3215.
20. Joo YK, Black EM, Trier I, Haakma W, Zou L, Kabeche L. ATR promotes clearance of damaged DNA and damaged cells by rupturing micronuclei. Mol Cell. 2023;83(20):3642–58 e3644. https://doi.org/10.1016/j.molcel.2023.09.003.
21. Karanam K, Kafri R, Loewer A, Lahav G. Quantitative live cell imaging reveals a gradual shift between DNA repair mechanisms and a maximal use of HR in mid S phase. Mol Cell. 2012;47(2):320–9. https://doi.org/10.1016/j.molcel.2012.05.052.
22. Kornepati AVR, Boyd JT, Murray CE, Saifetiarova J, de la Pena Avalos B, Rogers CM, Bai H, Padron AS, Liao Y, Ontiveros C, Svatek RS, Hromas R, Li R, Hu Y, Conejo-Garcia JR, Vadlamudi RK, Zhao W, Dray E, Sung P, Curiel TJ. Tumor intrinsic PD-L1 promotes DNA repair in distinct cancers and suppresses PARP inhibitor-induced synthetic lethality. Cancer Res. 2022;82(11):2156–70. https://doi.org/10.1158/0008-5472.CAN-21-2076.
23. Kovacs MT, Vallette M, Wiertsema P, Dingli F, Loew D, Nader GPF, Piel M, Ceccaldi R. DNA damage induces nuclear envelope rupture through ATR-mediated phosphorylation of lamin A/C. Mol Cell. 2023;83(20):3659–3668 e3610. https://doi.org/10.1016/j.molcel.2023.09.023.
24. Lee SJ, Jang BC, Lee SW, Yang YI, Suh SI, Park YM, Oh S, Shin JG, Yao S, Chen L, Choi IH. Interferon regulatory factor-1 is prerequisite to the constitutive expression and IFN-gamma-induced upregulation of B7-H1 (CD274). FEBS Lett. 2006;580(3):755–62. https://doi.org/10.1016/j.febslet.2005.12.093.

25. Li L, Yu R, Cai T, Chen Z, Lan M, Zou T, Wang B, Wang Q, Zhao Y, Cai Y. Effects of immune cells and cytokines on inflammation and immunosuppression in the tumor microenvironment. Int Immunopharmacol. 2020;88:106939. https://doi.org/10.1016/j.intimp.2020.106939.
26. Liu Y, Yang Z, Wang S, Miao R, Chang CM, Zhang J, Zhang X, Hung MC, Hou J. Nuclear PD-L1 compartmentalization suppresses tumorigenesis and overcomes immunocheckpoint therapy resistance in mice via histone macroH2A1. J Clin Invest. 2024;134(22):e181314. https://doi.org/10.1172/JCI181314.
27. Liu YT, Sun ZJ. Turning cold tumors into hot tumors by improving T-cell infiltration. Theranostics. 2021;11(11):5365–86. https://doi.org/10.7150/thno.58390.
28. Mackenzie KJ, Carroll P, Martin CA, Murina O, Fluteau A, Simpson DJ, Olova N, Sutcliffe H, Rainger JK, Leitch A, Osborn RT, Wheeler AP, Nowotny M, Gilbert N, Chandra T, Reijns MAM, Jackson AP. cGAS surveillance of micronuclei links genome instability to innate immunity. Nature. 2017;548(7668):461–5. https://doi.org/10.1038/nature23449.
29. Mimura K, Teh JL, Okayama H, Shiraishi K, Kua LF, Koh V, Smoot DT, Ashktorab H, Oike T, Suzuki Y, Fazreen Z, Asuncion BR, Shabbir A, Yong WP, So J, Soong R, Kono K. PD-L1 expression is mainly regulated by interferon gamma associated with JAK-STAT pathway in gastric cancer. Cancer Sci. 2018;109(1):43–53. https://doi.org/10.1111/cas.13424.
30. Moon JW, Kong SK, Kim BS, Kim HJ, Lim H, Noh K, Kim Y, Choi JW, Lee JH, Kim YS. IFNgamma induces PD-L1 overexpression by JAK2/STAT1/IRF-1 signaling in EBV-positive gastric carcinoma. Sci Rep. 2017;7(1):17810. https://doi.org/10.1038/s41598-017-18132-0.
31. Mukai K, Konno H, Akiba T, Uemura T, Waguri S, Kobayashi T, Barber GN, Arai H, Taguchi T. Activation of STING requires palmitoylation at the Golgi. Nat Commun. 2016;7:11932. https://doi.org/10.1038/ncomms11932.
32. Nihira NT, Wu W, Hosoi M, Togashi Y, Sunada S, Miyoshi Y, Miki Y, Ohta T. Nuclear PD-L1 triggers tumour-associated inflammation upon DNA damage. EMBO Rep. 2025;26(3):635–55. https://doi.org/10.1038/s44319-024-00354-9.
33. Pan BS, Perera SA, Piesvaux JA, Presland JP, Schroeder GK, Cumming JN, Trotter BW, Altman MD, Buevich AV, Cash B, Cemerski S, Chang W, Chen Y, Dandliker PJ, Feng G, Haidle A, Henderson T, Jewell J, Kariv I, Knemeyer I, Kopinja J, Lacey BM, Laskey J, Lesburg CA, Liang R, Long BJ, Lu M, Ma Y, Minnihan EC, O'Donnell G, Otte R, Price L, Rakhilina L, Sauvagnat B, Sharma S, Tyagarajan S, Woo H, Wyss DF, Xu S, Bennett DJ, Addona GH. An orally available non-nucleotide STING agonist with antitumor activity. Science. 2020;369(6506):eaba6098. https://doi.org/10.1126/science.aba6098.
34. Patel RS, Romero R, Watson EV, Liang AC, Burger M, Westcott PMK, Mercer KL, Bronson RT, Wooten EC, Bhutkar A, Jacks T, Elledge SJ. A GATA4-regulated secretory program suppresses tumors through recruitment of cytotoxic CD8 T cells. Nat Commun. 2022;13(1):256. https://doi.org/10.1038/s41467-021-27731-5.
35. Sasidharan Nair V, Toor SM, Ali BR, Elkord E. Dual inhibition of STAT1 and STAT3 activation downregulates expression of PD-L1 in human breast cancer cells. Expert Opin Ther Targets. 2018;22(6):547–57. https://doi.org/10.1080/14728222.2018.1471137.
36. Sato H, Niimi A, Yasuhara T, Permata TBM, Hagiwara Y, Isono M, Nuryadi E, Sekine R, Oike T, Kakoti S, Yoshimoto Y, Held KD, Suzuki Y, Kono K, Miyagawa K, Nakano T, Shibata A. DNA double-strand break repair pathway regulates PD-L1 expression in cancer cells. Nat Commun. 2017;8(1):1751. https://doi.org/10.1038/s41467-017-01883-9.
37. Schmid P, Adams S, Rugo HS, Schneeweiss A, Barrios CH, Iwata H, Dieras V, Hegg R, Im SA, Shaw Wright G, Henschel V, Molinero L, Chui SY, Funke R, Husain A, Winer EP, Loi S, Emens LA, IMpassion130 Trial Investigators. Atezolizumab and nab-paclitaxel in advanced triple-negative breast cancer. N Engl J Med. 2018;379(22):2108–21. https://doi.org/10.1056/NEJMoa1809615.
38. Schmid P, Dent R, O'Shaughnessy J. Pembrolizumab for early triple-negative breast cancer. Reply. N Engl J Med. 2020;382(26):e108. https://doi.org/10.1056/NEJMc2006684.

39. Schoonen PM, Talens F, Stok C, Gogola E, Heijink AM, Bouwman P, Foijer F, Tarsounas M, Blatter S, Jonkers J, Rottenberg S, van Vugt M. Progression through mitosis promotes PARP inhibitor-induced cytotoxicity in homologous recombination-deficient cancer cells. Nat Commun. 2017;8:15981. https://doi.org/10.1038/ncomms15981.
40. Shen J, Zhao W, Ju Z, Wang L, Peng Y, Labrie M, Yap TA, Mills GB, Peng G. PARPi triggers the STING-dependent immune response and enhances the therapeutic efficacy of immune checkpoint blockade independent of BRCAness. Cancer Res. 2019;79(2):311–9. https://doi.org/10.1158/0008-5472.CAN-18-1003.
41. Silver DP, Livingston DM. Mechanisms of BRCA1 tumor suppression. Cancer Discov. 2012;2(8):679–84. https://doi.org/10.1158/2159-8290.CD-12-0221.
42. Takahashi H, Behbakht K, McGovern PE, Chiu HC, Couch FJ, Weber BL, Friedman LS, King MC, Furusato M, LiVolsi VA, et al. Mutation analysis of the BRCA1 gene in ovarian cancers. Cancer Res. 1995;55(14):2998–3002. https://www.ncbi.nlm.nih.gov/pubmed/7606717.
43. Wang L, Geng H, Liu Y, Liu L, Chen Y, Wu F, Liu Z, Ling S, Wang Y, Zhou L. Hot and cold tumors: immunological features and the therapeutic strategies. MedComm (2020). 2023;4(5):e343. https://doi.org/10.1002/mco2.343.
44. Wang X, Li Y, Tang Y, Liu Z, Liu Y, Fu X, Guo S, Ma J, Ma F, Zhu Z, Zhang W, Ye L. PD-L1 delactylation-promoted nuclear translocation accelerates liver cancer growth through elevating SQLE transcription activity. Cancer Lett. 2025;630:217901. https://doi.org/10.1016/j.canlet.2025.217901.
45. Wen WX, Leong CO. Association of BRCA1- and BRCA2-deficiency with mutation burden, expression of PD-L1/PD-1, immune infiltrates, and T cell-inflamed signature in breast cancer. PLoS One. 2019;14(4):e0215381. https://doi.org/10.1371/journal.pone.0215381.
46. Zhou S, Liang Y, Hao Y, Wang Q, Xu Y, Su T, Cheng F, Zhu G. Combined cancer immunotherapy with lipid nanoparticle delivery of oligo-based cGAS-agonistic adjuvant and peptide or mRNA vaccines. Mol Ther Nucleic Acids. 2025;36(3):102623. https://doi.org/10.1016/j.omtn.2025.102623.

Tissue-Specific Carcinogenesis Induced by BRCA1 Deficiency

Yuki Yoshino, Zhenzhou Fang, and Natsuko Chiba

Abstract Germline pathogenic variants in *BRCA1 and BRCA2 (BRCA1/2)* cause hereditary breast and ovarian cancer syndrome (HBOC). The function of BRCA1/2 in homologous recombination (HR) repair is considered essential for their activity as tumor suppressors. At the same time, BRCA1/2 also contributes to multiple cellular processes, including the regulation of the centrosome. However, it remains unclear how the dysregulation of BRCA1/2 leads to tissue-specific carcinogenesis. Previously, we identified BRCA1-interacting proteins, Obg-like ATPase 1 (OLA1) and the receptor for activated C kinase 1 (RACK1), which function together with BRCA1 to regulate the number of centrosomes.

In this chapter, we describe the possible mechanisms that cause tissue-specific carcinogenesis in the breasts and ovaries of women with BRCA1 deficiency. We found that the characteristics of centrosome duplication in mammary cells and the effect of estrogen stimulation on centrosome amplification induced by OLA1 deficiency. These regulatory mechanisms of centrosome number may increase the risk of breast and ovarian cancers in individuals with *BRCA1* pathogenic variants.

Keywords Hereditary breast and ovarian cancer (HBOC) · BRCA1 · Centrosome · Estrogen · Tissue-specific carcinogenesis

---

Y. Yoshino · N. Chiba (✉)
Department of Cancer Biology, Institute of Development, Aging and Cancer (IDAC), Tohoku University, Aoba-ku, Sendai, Japan

Laboratory of Cancer Biology, Graduate School of Life Sciences, Tohoku University, Aoba-ku, Sendai, Japan

Department of Cancer Biology, Tohoku University Graduate School of Medicine, Aoba-ku, Sendai, Japan
e-mail: yuki.yoshino.c8@tohoku.ac.jp; natsuko.chiba.c7@tohoku.ac.jp

Z. Fang
Department of Cancer Biology, Institute of Development, Aging and Cancer (IDAC), Tohoku University, Aoba-ku, Sendai, Japan

Laboratory of Cancer Biology, Graduate School of Life Sciences, Tohoku University, Aoba-ku, Sendai, Japan

M. Arai et al. (eds.), *Practical Guide to Hereditary Breast and Ovarian Cancer IV*,
https://doi.org/10.1007/978-981-95-6580-1_2

1 Introduction

Germline alterations of *Breast Cancer Gene 1 (BRCA1)* cause hereditary breast and ovarian cancer syndrome (HBOC) [1]. BRCA1 forms complexes with BRCA1-associated RING domain 1 (BARD1) and other proteins to contribute to various cellular functions to maintain genome stability, including homologous recombination repair, centrosome regulation, transcription, chromatin remodeling, and stabilization of replication forks [2]. However, it remains unclear how the dysregulation of BRCA1 function leads to tissue-specific carcinogenesis.

Centrosomes are the primary microtubule (MT)-organizing centers (MTOCs) in animal cells, controlling cell shape, polarity, and motility and mediating bipolar spindle formation during mitosis [3, 4]. Centrosome consists of a pair of centrioles, the mother and daughter centrioles, surrounded by the pericentriolar matrix (PCM) (Fig. 1a). The single centrosome in the G1 phase duplicates only once per cell cycle. Centrosome duplication is governed by centriole duplication during the cell cycle (Fig. 1b). Centriole duplication is initiated by the separation of a pair of centrioles (centriole disengagement) in the late mitosis-early G1 phase. The new daughter centrioles form a procentriole perpendicular to two centrioles in early S phase. Each daughter centriole elongates during the S and G2 phases. During the G2 and M phases, the amount of PCM proteins increases (centrosome maturation), enhancing the ability to nucleate and anchor microtubules. The two centrosomes separate in the late G2 phase, migrate to form the two opposing poles of the mitotic spindle, and function in proper segregation of chromosomes in mitosis to maintain genome stability [5].

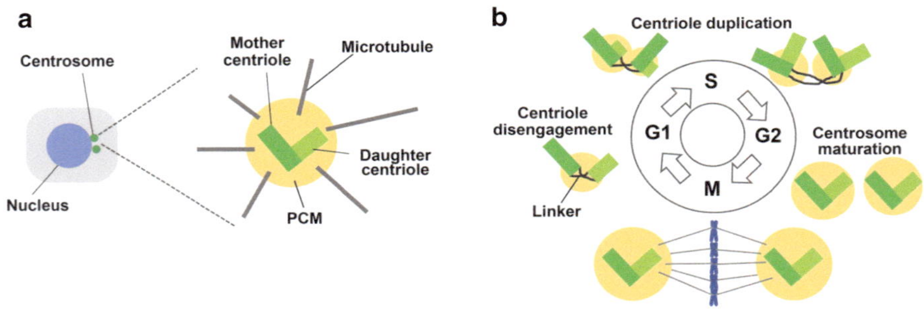

Fig. 1 Structure and duplication of the centrosome. (**a**) Structure of the centrosome. The centrosome consists of a pair of mother and daughter centrioles, embedded in the pericentriolar matrix (PCM). The PCM plays roles in nucleating, anchoring, and positioning microtubules. (**b**) Centrosome duplication in the cell cycle. The mother and daughter centrioles are disengaged in the late mitosis-early G1 phase. After centriole disengagement, a proteinaceous linker forms between the two centrioles, connecting them. The building of the new centriole begins in the early S phase by the formation of a procentriole at each centriole. One new daughter centriole is created for each mother centriole during the S and G2 phases. In the G2 phase, the size of the centrosome increases by the recruitment of PCM proteins. In the late G2 phase, the two centrosomes separate through the dissolution of the linker and move to opposite sides of the cell to form the spindle poles

Aberrations of centrosome number and structure are frequently observed in various cancers [6]. Centrosome amplification can lead to chromosome segregation errors and is linked to the invasive phenotype of cancers, contributing to carcinogenesis and cancer progression [7, 8].

Previously, we identified BRCA1-interacting proteins, Obg-like ATPase 1 (OLA1) and the receptor for activated C kinase 1 (RACK1), which function to regulate the number of centrosomes together with BRCA1 and BARD1 [9, 10]. We revealed that alterations in these BRCA1-interacting proteins cause centrosome amplification in mammary tissue-derived cells [9–13]. Here, we describe possible mechanisms of tissue-specific carcinogenesis caused by the dysregulation of centrosome number, which is controlled by BRCA1-interacting proteins.

2 Characteristics of Centriole Duplication in Mammary Tissue-Derived Cells Contribute to the Tissue-Specific Carcinogenesis by Alterations in BRCA1-Interacting Proteins

BRCA1 and BARD1 have a RING domain at their amino (N)-terminal region1 and two BRCT domains at the carboxy (C)-terminal region [2, 12, 13]. BRCA1 and BARD1 form a heterodimer via their RING domains [14]. We identified OLA1 as a protein that interacts with the C-terminal region of BARD1 [9]. OLA1 is a member of the YchF subfamily of Obg-like GTPases and is highly conserved from yeast to humans [15–17]. OLA is overexpressed in many malignancies [18]. OLA1 directly binds to the N-terminal region of BRCA1, the C-terminal region of BARD1, and an essential PCM protein, γ-tubulin (Fig. 2) [9]. OLA1 interacts with the middle portion of BRCA1 via γ-tubulin and the C-terminal region of BRCA1 [9]. OLA1 localizes to the centrosome throughout the cell cycle; however, its centrosomal localization decreases in the G2 phase [19]. We revealed that Aurora A, which is a critical kinase that functions in centrosome maturation and bipolar spindle assembly, polyubiquitinates OLA1 as an E3 ubiquitin ligase (E3), targeting it for proteasomal degradation in the G2 phase [19, 20]. The reduction of centrosomal localization of OLA1 by the E3 activity of Aurora A contributes to centrosome maturation [19].

Furthermore, we identified the receptor for activated C kinase (RACK1) as a protein that interacts with OLA1 [10]. RACK1 is also highly conserved from yeast to humans and is composed of seven Trp-Asp (WD) domains. RACK1 functions as a scaffolding protein in various cellular processes, including cell motility, proliferation, cell survival and death, and tumorigenesis [21]. RACK1 binds to BRCA1, OLA1, and γ-tubulin, is associated with BARD1, and localizes to centrosomes in interphase and spindle poles in mitosis. RACK1 is involved in the centrosomal localization of BRCA1 in interphase [10].

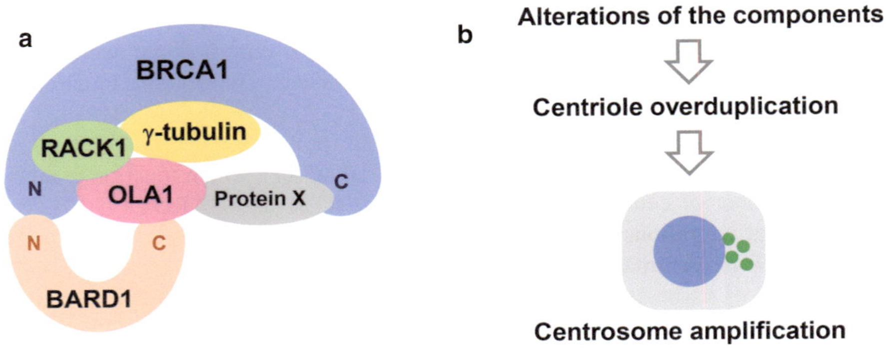

Fig. 2 BRCA1/BARD1/OLA1/RACK1 complex. (**a**) BRCA1 and BARD1 bind to each other via their RING domains in their N-terminal regions. OLA1 binds to the N-terminal region of BRCA1, the C-terminal region of BARD1, and γ-tubulin. The middle region of BRCA1 binds to γ-tubulin and interacts with OLA1 via γ-tubulin. The C-terminal region of BRCA1 may be associated with OLA1 via an unknown protein, Protein X. RACK1 binds to the N-terminal region of BRCA1, OLA1, and γ-tubulin and is associated with BARD1. "N" indicates the N-terminus of the protein. "C" indicates the C-terminus of the protein. (**b**) Alterations in the components of the BRCA1/BARD1/OLA1/RACK1 complex, such as abnormal expression and cancer-associated mutations, cause centriole duplication, leading to centrosome amplification

Aberrant expressions and cancer-associated variants of BRCA1, BARD1, OLA1, and RACK1 cause centrosome amplification in mammary tissue-derived cells, but not in non-mammary tissue-derived cells. The suppression of BRCA1 or OLA1 and the overexpression of OLA1 or RACK1 cause centriole overduplication, leading to centrosome amplification [9–13, 22–24]. Therefore, we presumed that centrosomes in mammary cells possess specific characteristics that facilitate the induction of centrosome amplification by dysregulation of centrosome duplication. Consistent with our hypothesis, immunostaining for the centrosome with an anti-γ-tubulin antibody and the centriole with an anti-centrin antibody in mammary tissue-derived cells revealed that most cells with two γ-tubulin foci contained more than two centrioles. By contrast, in other tissue-derived cells, more than half of the cells with two γ-tubulin foci included two centrioles [10]. These results indicate that the number of centrioles is higher in mammary cells than in those derived from other tissues. Although the mechanisms have not been elucidated yet, they may be attributed to an earlier timing of centriole duplication or increased efficiency of centriole duplication. Therefore, mammary cells might be sensitive to centriole overduplication induced by alterations of BRCA1, BARD1, OLA1, or RACK1, resulting in centrosome amplification. We presume that these characteristics of centrosome duplication in mammary tissue-derived cells contribute to the tissue-specific carcinogenesis in mammary tissues induced by *BRCA1* germline pathogenic variants.

3 Estrogen Stimulation Is Involved in Carcinogenesis in *Ola1*-Knockout Mice

3.1 Knockout of **Ola1** *in Female Mice Induces Tumors with Centrosome Amplification*

We deleted exon 3 in the *Ola1* gene by conventional gene targeting with the Cre/lox system to generate *Ola1*-knockout mice and elucidate the role of Ola1 deficiency in tumorigenesis [25]. During intrauterine development, the percentage of *Ola1−/−* embryos was significantly lower than the expected ratios, suggesting that homozygous knockout of *Ola1* induced embryonic lethality in mice. There were no apparent differences morphologically and histologically between *Ola1+/−* and *Ola1+/+* embryos, whereas the *Ola1−/−* embryos were smaller than the *Ola1+/+* or *Ola1+/−* embryos and exhibited poor development of alveoli, bronchi, and hepatic ducts [25].

In addition, we found that some old *Ola1+/−* mice had enlarged spleens. Pathological investigation revealed three abnormal histological patterns in the spleen of *Ola1+/−* mice: malignant lymphoma, lymphoproliferation with atypical cells, and hyperplasia of hematopoietic cells. The frequency of lymphoproliferative disease, malignant lymphoma, and lymphoproliferation with atypical cells was markedly higher in Ola1+/− female mice than in male mice. Malignant lymphoma was found only in *Ola1+/−* female mice. Lymphoma cells were CD10- and CD20-positive, but CD3-negative, suggesting a B-cell lymphoma. Since OLA1 knockdown induces centrosome amplification in human cells, we stained malignant lymphoma, lymphoproliferation with atypical cells, and normal tissues with an antibody against γ-tubulin. The frequency of cells with centrosome amplification in malignant lymphoma was markedly higher than that in the other types, and the centrosome amplification frequency in lymphoproliferation with atypical cells was significantly higher than that in normal tissue in *Ola1+/−* mice. Furthermore, abnormal mitosis, including multipolar division, was frequently observed in malignant lymphoma [25].

Ola1 protein levels were analyzed by immunofluorescence staining with an anti-OLA1 antibody. The Ola1 intensity of the malignant lymphoma tissues was significantly lower than that of the normal tissues in *Ola1+/−* mice. Moreover, the Ola1 intensities in spleen tissues correlated negatively with the frequency of cells with centrosome amplification. These indicate that Ola1 deficiency causes centrosome amplification, leading to a malignant phenotype [25].

Next, we investigated the number of centrosomes in splenocytes from normal spleens of male and female mice. The frequency of splenocytes with centrosome amplification was higher in *Ola1+/−* mice than in *Ola1+/+* mice. Contrary to expectations, the frequency of splenocytes with centrosome amplification was significantly higher in male *Ola1+/−* mice than in female *Ola1+/−* mice [25].

3.2 Estrogen Stimulation Reduces Cells with Centrosome Amplification Induced by OLA1 Knockdown

We presumed that female hormones, estrogen and progesterone, might affect the tumorigenesis with centrosome amplification induced by Ola1 deficiency. We treated human cells with these hormones and analyzed the number of centrosomes. MCF7 and T47D are human breast cancer cell lines that express both estrogen receptor (ER) and progesterone receptor (PgR) [25]. We knocked down OLA1 in these cells and treated them with β-estradiol, a potent estrogen. β-Estradiol treatment moderately increased cells with centrosome amplification. OLA1 knockdown markedly increased the frequency of cells with centrosome amplification, as we reported previously [11]. Interestingly, β-estradiol treatment significantly inhibited OLA1 knockdown-induced centrosome amplification to the level treated only with β-estradiol. By contrast, treatment with medroxyprogesterone acetate did not affect the number of centrosomes in control or OLA1-knockdown MCF7 cells [25]. These findings suggest that PgR signaling is not involved in regulating the number of centrosomes.

β-Estradiol treatment did not increase the cells with centrosome amplification in Hs578T and MDA-MB-231 cells, which do not express ER. These suggest that the ER is required for the regulation of centrosome amplification. OLA1 knockdown induces centrosome amplification in MDA-MB-231 and Hs578T cells. However, both β-estradiol treatment and expression of FLAG-ERα are required for the reduction of cells with centrosome amplification induced by OLA1 knockdown [25].

3.3 Model of Tumorigenesis in Female Ola1+/− Mice

Although most lymphoproliferative diseases were observed in *Ola1+/−* female mice, centrosome amplification was more frequently found in splenocytes from the normal spleen in male *Ola1+/−* mice. Treatment with estrogen suppressed centrosome amplification induced by OLA1-knockdown cells expressing ERα. Therefore, estrogen stimulation, mediated by ERα, suppresses centrosome amplification induced by OLA1 deficiency.

Polo-like kinase 4 (PLK4) plays a critical role in the initiation of centriole duplication, and overexpression of PLK4 causes centriole duplication, resulting in centrosome amplification [26]. Several mouse models that overexpress Plk4 have been developed to analyze carcinogenesis induced by centrosome amplification [27–32]. A mouse model that moderately overexpresses Plk4 by a doxycycline-inducible system resulted in tumorigenesis [27]. However, mice models created by the integration of Cre-inducible *Plk4* transgenes to overexpress Plk4 caused centrosome amplification, but not in tumorigenesis [28, 29, 32]. Since severe centrosome amplification induces aberrant mitosis resulting in mitotic cell death, prominent centrosome amplification might disturb the survival of pre-malignant cells and prevent

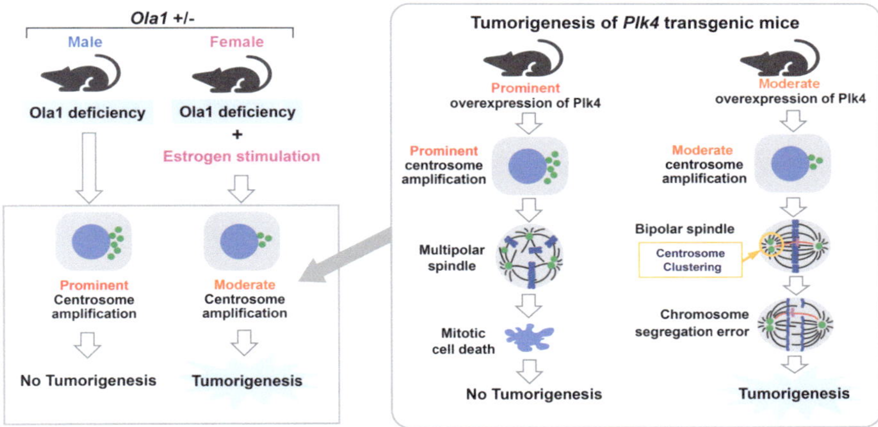

Fig. 3 A schematic image of tumorigenesis in female *Ola1*+/− mice. In male *Ola1*+/− mice, *Ola1* deficiency leads to prominent centrosome amplification in cells, resulting in aberrant mitosis and subsequent mitotic cell death. In female *Ola1*+/− mice, centrosome amplification was moderate compared to that in male *Ola1*+/− mice. We found that estrogen stimulation partially suppresses centrosome amplification induced by the knockdown of OLA1 in deficiency. Mouse models that overexpress Plk4 revealed that moderate overexpression of Plk4 is more tumorigenic than prominent overexpression of Plk4. We presume that cells with moderate centrosome amplification can form bipolar spindles by centrosome clustering and complete mitosis. However, these cells could acquire chromosomal instability due to chromosome missegregation, which promotes tumorigenesis

carcinogenesis. However, moderate centrosome amplification may allow the survival of pre-malignant cells, as they can proceed through mitosis via centrosome clustering.

Taken together, these findings suggest that moderate centrosome amplification induced by Ola1 deficiency and estrogen stimulation in female Ola1+/− mice is more tumorigenic than the prominent centrosome amplification induced by *Ola1* deficiency alone in male *Ola1*+/− mice (Fig. 3). Therefore, estrogen stimulation in female *Ola1*+/− mice, which suppresses centrosome amplification to a moderate level in cells with Ola1 insufficiency, increases the chances of survival in pre-malignant cells, thereby contributing to carcinogenesis. We presume that this function of estrogen stimulation contributes to estrogen-sensitive tissue carcinogenesis in the breasts and ovaries of women.

4 Conclusions

Although BRCA1 is involved in multiple cellular processes, the role of BRCA1 alterations in the mechanisms underlying tissue-specific carcinogenesis remains unclear. We identified the characteristics of centrosome duplication, enhanced efficiency of centriole duplication, in mammary tissue-derived cells. Furthermore, we revealed that estrogen stimulation reduces centrosome amplification induced by BRCA1-associated protein deficiency; however, moderate centrosome amplification contributes to carcinogenesis in estrogen-sensitive tissues. We presume that these mechanisms are combined and cause the high risk of breast and ovarian cancers by *BRCA1* germline pathogenic variants. Interestingly, BRCA2 also localizes to centrosomes and is involved in centriole duplication [33, 34]. These mechanisms may also contribute to carcinogenesis through alterations in the *BRCA2* gene.

References

1. Miki Y, Swensen J, Shattuck-Eidens D, Futreal PA, Harshman K, Tavtigian S, et al. A strong candidate for the breast and ovarian cancer susceptibility gene BRCA1. Science. 1994;266(5182):66–71.
2. Takaoka M, Miki Y. BRCA1 gene: function and deficiency. Int J Clin Oncol. 2018;23(1):36–44.
3. Conduit PT, Wainman A, Raff JW. Centrosome function and assembly in animal cells. Nat Rev Mol Cell Biol. 2015;16(10):611–24.
4. Nigg EA, Holland AJ. Once and only once: mechanisms of centriole duplication and their deregulation in disease. Nat Rev Mol Cell Biol. 2018;19(5):297–312.
5. Fujita H, Yoshino Y, Chiba N. Regulation of the centrosome cycle. Mol Cell Oncol. 2016;3(2):e1075643.
6. Nigg EA, Schnerch D, Ganier O. Impact of centrosome aberrations on chromosome segregation and tissue architecture in cancer. Cold Spring Harb Symp Quant Biol. 2017;82:137–44.
7. Gonczy P. Centrosomes and cancer: revisiting a long-standing relationship. Nat Rev Cancer. 2015;15(11):639–52.
8. Godinho SA, Picone R, Burute M, Dagher R, Su Y, Leung CT, et al. Oncogene-like induction of cellular invasion from centrosome amplification. Nature. 2014;510(7503):167–71.
9. Matsuzawa A, Kanno S, Nakayama M, Mochiduki H, Wei L, Shimaoka T, et al. The BRCA1/BARD1-interacting protein OLA1 functions in centrosome regulation. Mol Cell. 2014;53(1):101–14.
10. Yoshino Y, Qi H, Kanazawa R, Sugamata M, Suzuki K, Kobayashi A, et al. RACK1 regulates centriole duplication by controlling localization of BRCA1 to the centrosome in mammary tissue-derived cells. Oncogene. 2019;38(16):3077–92.
11. Yoshino Y, Qi H, Fujita H, Shirota M, Abe S, Komiyama Y, et al. BRCA1-interacting protein OLA1 requires interaction with BARD1 to regulate centrosome number. Mol Cancer Res. 2018;16:1499.
12. Otsuka K, Yoshino Y, Qi H, Chiba N. The function of BARD1 in centrosome regulation in cooperation with BRCA1/OLA1/RACK1. Genes (Basel). 2020;11(8):842.
13. Yoshino Y, Fang Z, Qi H, Kobayashi A, Chiba N. Dysregulation of the centrosome induced by BRCA1 deficiency contributes to tissue-specific carcinogenesis. Cancer Sci. 2021;112:1679.
14. Brzovic PS, Keeffe JR, Nishikawa H, Miyamoto K, Fox D 3rd, Fukuda M, et al. Binding and recognition in the assembly of an active BRCA1/BARD1 ubiquitin-ligase complex. Proc Natl Acad Sci USA. 2003;100(10):5646–51.
15. Verstraeten N, Fauvart M, Versees W, Michiels J. The universally conserved prokaryotic GTPases. Microbiol Mol Biol Rev. 2011;75(3):507–42, second and third pages of table of contents.
16. Leipe DD, Wolf YI, Koonin EV, Aravind L. Classification and evolution of P-loop GTPases and related ATPases. J Mol Biol. 2002;317(1):41–72.

17. Teplyakov A, Obmolova G, Chu SY, Toedt J, Eisenstein E, Howard AJ, et al. Crystal structure of the YchF protein reveals binding sites for GTP and nucleic acid. J Bacteriol. 2003;185(14):4031–7.
18. Sun H, Luo X, Montalbano J, Jin W, Shi J, Sheikh MS, et al. DOC45, a novel DNA damage-regulated nucleocytoplasmic ATPase that is overexpressed in multiple human malignancies. Mol Cancer Res. 2010;8(1):57–66.
19. Fang Z, Li X, Yoshino Y, Suzuki M, Qi H, Murooka H, et al. Aurora A polyubiquitinates the BRCA1-interacting protein OLA1 to promote centrosome maturation. Cell Rep. 2023;42(8):112850.
20. Fang Z, Li X, Yoshino Y, Chiba N. Protocol to detect OLA1 polyubiquitination by Aurora A in vivo and in vitro. STAR Protoc. 2024;5(2):103008.
21. Adams DR, Ron D, Kiely PA. RACK1, A multifaceted scaffolding protein: structure and function. Cell Commun Signal. 2011;9:22.
22. Starita LM, Machida Y, Sankaran S, Elias JE, Griffin K, Schlegel BP, et al. BRCA1-dependent ubiquitination of gamma-tubulin regulates centrosome number. Mol Cell Biol. 2004;24(19):8457–66.
23. Ko MJ, Murata K, Hwang DS, Parvin JD. Inhibition of BRCA1 in breast cell lines causes the centrosome duplication cycle to be disconnected from the cell cycle. Oncogene. 2006;25(2):298–303.
24. Kais Z, Parvin JD. Regulation of centrosomes by the BRCA1-dependent ubiquitin ligase. Cancer Biol Ther. 2008;7(10):1540–3.
25. Yoshino Y, Ogoh H, Iichi Y, Sasaki T, Yoshida T, Ichimura S, et al. Knockout of Brca1-interacting factor Ola1 in female mice induces tumors with estrogen suppressible centrosome amplification. Biochim Biophys Acta Mol basis Dis. 2024;1870(5):167138.
26. Kleylein-Sohn J, Westendorf J, Le Clech M, Habedanck R, Stierhof YD, Nigg EA. Plk4-induced centriole biogenesis in human cells. Dev Cell. 2007;13(2):190–202.
27. Levine MS, Bakker B, Boeckx B, Moyett J, Lu J, Vitre B, et al. Centrosome amplification is sufficient to promote spontaneous tumorigenesis in mammals. Dev Cell. 2017;40(3):313–22 e5.
28. Sercin O, Larsimont JC, Karambelas AE, Marthiens V, Moers V, Boeckx B, et al. Transient PLK4 overexpression accelerates tumorigenesis in p53-deficient epidermis. Nat Cell Biol. 2016;18(1):100–10.
29. Vitre B, Holland AJ, Kulukian A, Shoshani O, Hirai M, Wang Y, et al. Chronic centrosome amplification without tumorigenesis. Proc Natl Acad Sci USA. 2015;112(46):E6321–30.
30. Coelho PA, Bury L, Shahbazi MN, Liakath-Ali K, Tate PH, Wormald S, et al. Over-expression of Plk4 induces centrosome amplification, loss of primary cilia and associated tissue hyperplasia in the mouse. Open Biol. 2015;5(12):150209.
31. Marthiens V, Rujano MA, Pennetier C, Tessier S, Paul-Gilloteaux P, Basto R. Centrosome amplification causes microcephaly. Nat Cell Biol. 2013;15(7):731–40.
32. Kulukian A, Holland AJ, Vitre B, Naik S, Cleveland DW, Fuchs E. Epidermal development, growth control, and homeostasis in the face of centrosome amplification. Proc Natl Acad Sci USA. 2015;112(46):E6311–20.
33. Nakanishi A, Han X, Saito H, Taguchi K, Ohta Y, Imajoh-Ohmi S, et al. Interference with BRCA2, which localizes to the centrosome during S and early M phase, leads to abnormal nuclear division. Biochem Biophys Res Commun. 2007;355(1):34–40.
34. Han X, Saito H, Miki Y, Nakanishi A. A CRM1-mediated nuclear export signal governs cytoplasmic localization of BRCA2 and is essential for centrosomal localization of BRCA2. Oncogene. 2008;27(21):2969–77.

Advances in Genetics

BRCA1/2 Pathogenic Variant-Based Precision Cancer Medicine: Insights Obtained from Real-World C-CAT Data

Takashi Kohno

Abstract Since 2019, comprehensive genomic profiling (CGP) has been implemented in Japan under the national health insurance system, and the resulting data have been aggregated systematically at the Center for Cancer Genomics and Advanced Therapeutics (C-CAT). To date, genomic and clinical information has been collected from more than 100,000 patients with solid tumors, providing an invaluable nationwide real-world data resource. Among 105,940 patients, 4383 (4.1%) harbored pathogenic variants of *BRCA1/2*, most commonly in breast, prostate, pancreatic, and ovarian cancers. Comparison with an international dataset revealed Japan-specific hotspot mutations such as *BRCA1* L63* and *BRCA2* R2318*. Importantly, there was a marked change in treatment approaches for patients with BRCA1/2 pathogenic variants. Before CGP testing, cytotoxic chemotherapies predominated; however, after CGP testing, the main treatment was Olaparib, a PARP inhibitor. This change in approach reflects clinical adoption of synthetic lethality-based treatments. Combining large-scale CGP data with clinical information can provide critical insight into the implementation of precision cancer medicine in real-world practice.

Keywords *BRCA1* · *BRCA2* · Cancer genomic profiling (CGP) · C-CAT · Real-world data · Cancer precision medicine

1 Introduction

Since 2019, the Japanese national health insurance system has implemented comprehensive genomic profiling (CGP) tests (also referred to as cancer gene panel tests) for patients with advanced solid tumors who have completed, or are expected

T. Kohno (✉)
Center for Cancer Genomics and Advanced Therapeutics (C-CAT), National Cancer Center, Chuo-ku, Tokyo, Japan
e-mail: tkkohno@ncc.go.jp

M. Arai et al. (eds.), *Practical Guide to Hereditary Breast and Ovarian Cancer IV*,
https://doi.org/10.1007/978-981-95-6580-1_3

to complete, standard chemotherapy. After obtaining consent from patients who have undergone CGP testing, data are aggregated at the Center for Cancer Genomics and Advanced Therapeutics (C-CAT), established within the National Cancer Center, Japan [1]. By the end of March 2025, more than 100,000 patients with solid tumors will have undergone CGP testing (https://for-patients.c-cat.ncc.go.jp/registration_status/), and for each of them, C-CAT generates a “C-CAT Findings Report” that includes the clinical significance of identified genetic alterations and information about domestic clinical trials, all of which support clinical decision-making. Furthermore, extensive efforts by designated cancer genomic medicine hospitals nationwide mean that C-CAT receives not only data regarding genomic alterations, but also clinical information about the patients who underwent CGP. This article describes current C-CAT data, with a focus on *BRCA1* and *BRCA2* mutations, and then discusses the current status and future prospects of cancer genomic medicine in Japan.

2 Characteristics of Cancers Registered in C-CAT

Figure 1 shows the distribution of cancer types registered in C-CAT. The registry contains information about many intractable cancers, including pancreatic cancer and soft tissue sarcomas. In addition, cancers with a strong hereditary component, such as breast and ovarian cancers, are also frequently represented. Notably, the number of registered ovarian cancer cases is disproportionately higher than that of breast cancer cases, reflecting both the intractable nature of the former disease and the clinical need for treatment strategies based on hereditary predisposition. Although limited to approximately 50 cases, male breast cancer cases are also included, providing a valuable dataset.

Clinical information (summarized in Fig. 2) has been collected for all these patients in the form of structured data, including drug names, treatment start and end dates, treatment responses, and the presence of grade ≥3 adverse events. These datasets provide a valuable real-world resource that improves our understanding of both the current landscape and the longitudinal trends of cancer genomic medicine in Japan. Information about family history has also been collected, allowing insight into the management of hereditary tumors.

3 Utilization of C-CAT Data

More than 99% of patients whose data are submitted to C-CAT have consented to secondary use of their clinical and genomic information. This exceptionally high rate of consent likely reflects the strong trust built between patients and hospital staff in the clinical setting. As a result, the CGP-tested cohort can be studied with minimal selection bias, providing an authentic picture of cancer genomic medicine,

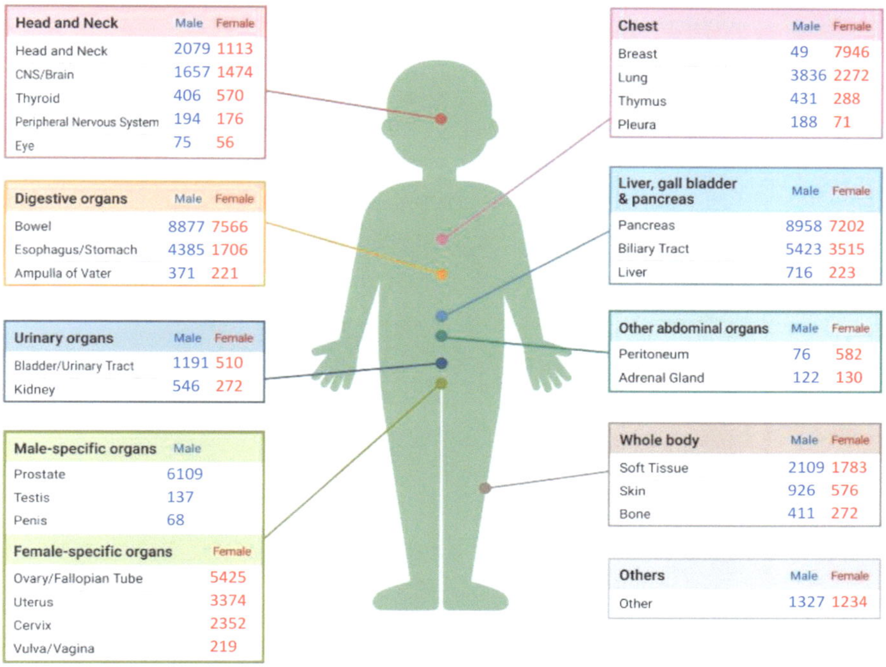

Fig. 1 Data registration in C-CAT by OncoTree classification. Summary as of June 12, 2025

while also facilitating academic research and drug development. Since the initiation of C-CAT data sharing in 2021, more than 100 groups, including 15 pharmaceutical companies, have accessed the data (https://www.ncc.go.jp/jp/c_cat/use/release/index.html). Specifically, C-CAT has launched the Research Use Portal, which allows users to securely access the data via their own computers using a two-factor authenticated internet connection. Importantly, all search results, as well as intellectual property derived from the analyses, belong entirely to the users. For example, the *KRAS* G12C mutation, which is a newly-identified and relatively rare druggable alteration [2] (slightly over 1% of all cases), has been observed across multiple cancer types, totaling as many as 1250 cases. Expert Panel recommendations following CGP testing show that sotorasib, a specific inhibitor of the KRAS G12C molecule, is the most frequently prescribed agent. Currently, sotorasib is approved only for lung cancer; however, broader indications across various cancers are anticipated, which will likely expand the distribution of therapies in the future.

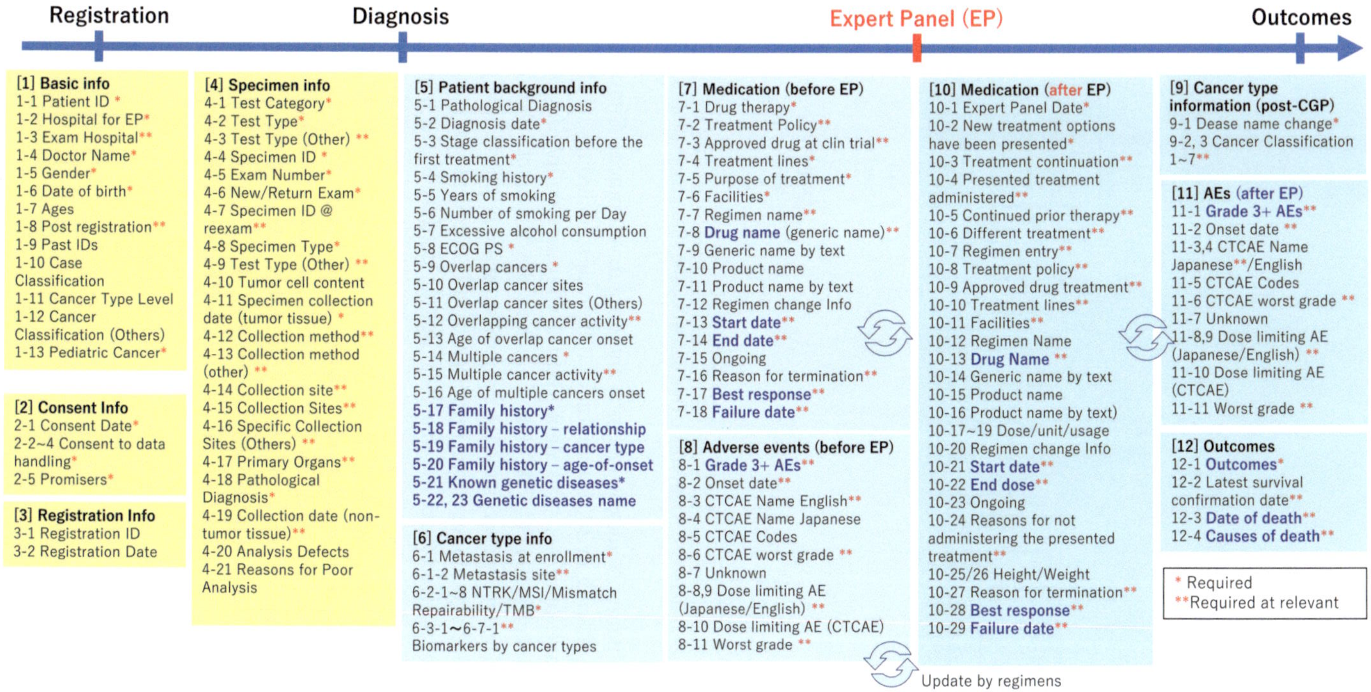

Fig. 2 Clinical information aggregated in C-CAT. Items mentioned in the text are shown in bold

4 Cancers Harboring Mutations in *BRCA1* and *BRCA2*

Figure 3 shows the results of a search for pathogenic variants of *BRCA1* and *BRCA2*. In total, 4383 patients harbored such alterations, accounting for 4.1% of 105,940 cases. Breast cancer was one of the most common cancer types, followed by prostate, pancreatic, and ovarian cancer, all of which are strongly associated with hereditary predisposition. Among the CGP tests covered by the national insurance system, FoundationOne CDx accounts for the largest number of cases, but does not distinguish between germline and somatic variants. Accordingly, the data presented here include both variants. Of particular note is the distribution of therapeutic agents. Before CGP testing, cytotoxic agents such as paclitaxel and carboplatin were commonly administered; however, after CGP testing, olaparib is the overwhelming first choice. This reflects the real-world practice of precision oncology using PARP inhibitors, which are synthetic lethality-based agents [3], based on CGP results in Japan.

Figure 4 shows pathogenic variants of *BRCA1* and *BRCA2* visualized as lollipop plots and compared with data from Project GENIE, a large-scale CGP database led by the American Association for Cancer Research [4] (Fig. 4). Japan-specific hotspot mutations such as BRCA1 L63* and BRCA2 R2318* [5] are strikingly common, indicating that the C-CAT database contains a substantial proportion of germline mutations. As more data from more cases are accumulated, it is anticipated that analyses will elucidate clinically relevant associations such as the relationship between variant positions, family history, and sensitivity to PARP inhibitors.

5 Conclusion

Analyses of C-CAT data have revealed the genetic characteristics of cancers in Japanese patients, leading to the publication of more than 50 peer-reviewed articles in international journals. In addition, although still limited, there are already cases in which pharmaceutical companies have utilized C-CAT data for regulatory approval of anticancer agents (https://www.ncc.go.jp/jp/c_cat/use/release/010/index.html). By contrast, studies specifically addressing germline variants, hereditary tumors, and cross-cancer-type investigations remain scarce. Under Japan's universal health insurance system, the collection of information about germline variants and the patients harboring them, as well as its application to clinical management of hereditary tumors, is of critical importance. We expect that future utilization of C-CAT data will generate impactful findings to advance this field of medicine.

Acknowledgments This study was supported by the National Cancer Center Research and Development Fund (2023-A-26).

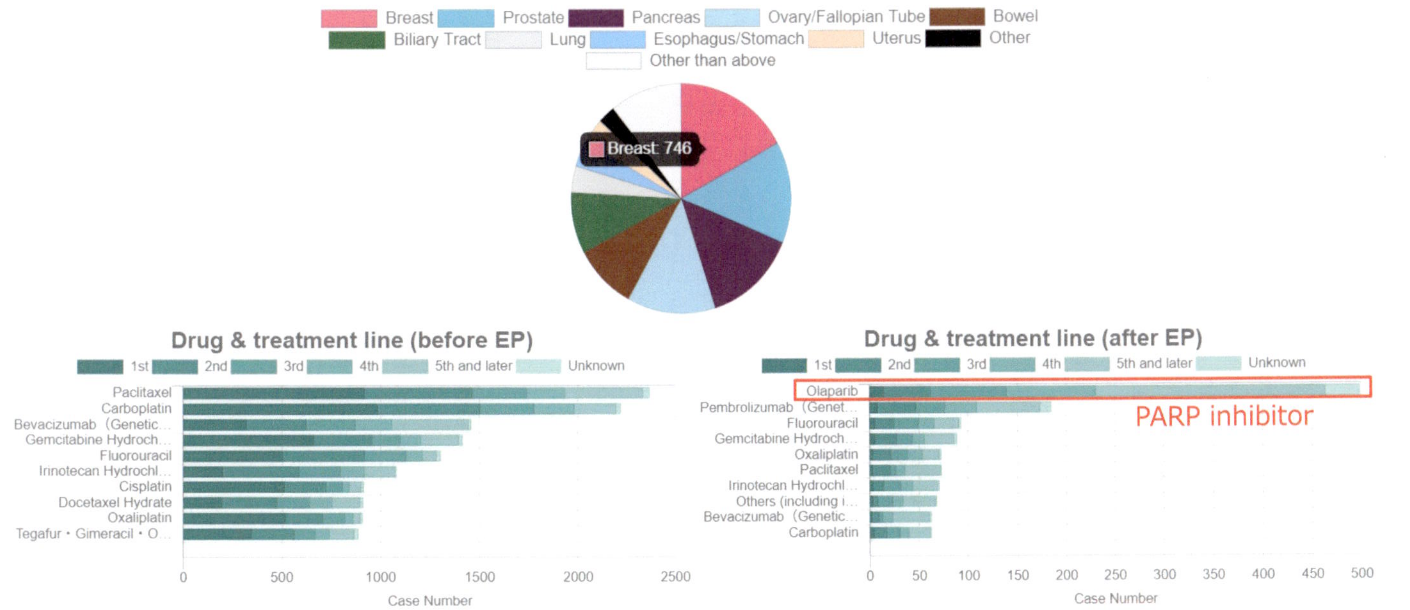

Fig. 3 Search results for pathogenic variants in *BRCA1* and *BRCA2* using the C-CAT Research Use Portal. Notably, olaparib, a PARP inhibitor, was the favored treatment after CGP testing

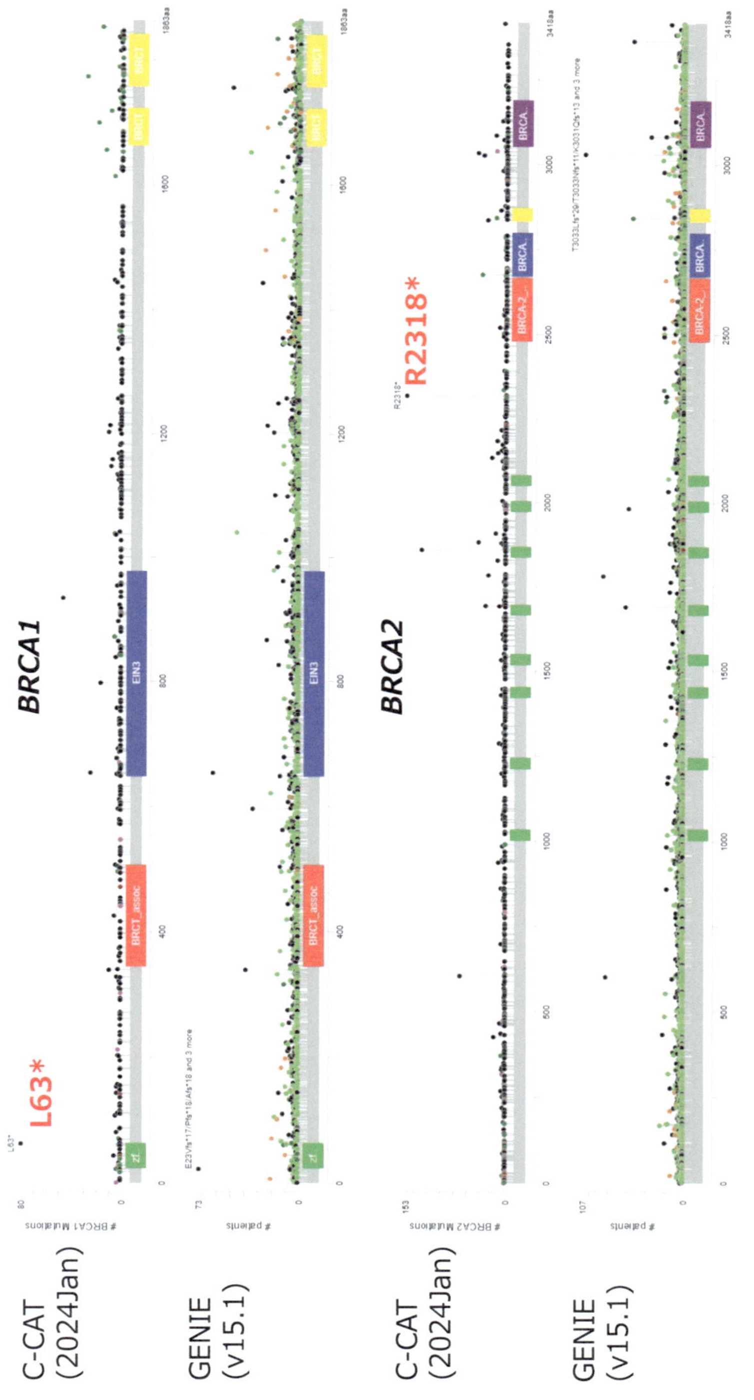

Fig. 4 Differences in the distribution of pathogenic variants of *BRCA1* and *BRCA2* between C-CAT and the U.S. Project GENIE datasets. Japanese-specific hotspot variants such as *BRCA1* L63* and *BRCA2* R2318* are highlighted

References

1. Kohno T, et al. C-CAT: the national datacenter for cancer genomic medicine in Japan. Cancer Discov. 2022;12:2509–15.
2. Vitiello PP, et al. KRAS G12C inhibition in solid tumors: biological breakthroughs, clinical evidence, and open challenges. Cancers (Basel). 2025;17:2803.
3. Gonçalves E, Ryan CJ, Adams DJ. Synthetic lethality in cancer drug discovery: challenges and opportunities. Nat Rev Drug Discov. 2025;25:22.
4. AACR Project GENIE Consortium. AACR Project GENIE: powering precision medicine through an international consortium. Cancer Discov. 2017;7:818–31.
5. Momozawa Y, et al. Expansion of cancer risk profile for BRCA1 and BRCA2 pathogenic variants. JAMA Oncol. 2022;8:871–8.

Translating Moderate-Risk Gene Data into Clinical Practice: Focus on *CHEK2* Germline Pathogenic Variants

Yuri Takehara and Yukihide Momozawa

Abstract *CHEK2* is one of the most frequently detected moderate-risk genes in multigene panel testing for cancer; however, its clinical utility remains limited, particularly outside of European populations. Especially, while previous studies have reported associations between *CHEK2* germline pathogenic variants (GPVs) and various cancers such as colorectal, prostate, renal, and thyroid, the evidence remains inconsistent. To address this gap and explore how to utilize data on *CHEK2* in clinical practice, particularly in Japan, we recently reported a large-scale case-control study in Japan using genome sequencing data from 112,141 individuals and functional analysis. We found significant associations between *CHEK2* GPVs and both female breast cancer (OR = 1.8, $P = 1.2 \times 10^{-3}$) and prostate cancer (OR = 1.8, $P = 1.7 \times 10^{-3}$). No significant differences were observed in age at diagnosis, tumor aggressiveness, or overall survival between GPV carriers and non-carriers. These findings suggest that *CHEK2* contributes similarly to cancer risk in Japanese and European populations. Our results are essential to support clinical decision-making and define appropriate management of *CHEK2* carriers in Japan.

Keywords *CHEK2* · Cancer genetics · Breast cancer · Prostate cancer

1 Background

Advances in next-generation sequencing have facilitated the widespread implementation of multigene panel testing for cancer, which is now expected to be covered by health insurance in Japan. It enables simultaneous assessment of multiple cancer-predisposition genes and identification of individuals carrying germline pathogenic variants (GPVs) in these genes. These findings can inform risk-reduction strategies

Y. Takehara · Y. Momozawa (✉)
Laboratory for Genotyping Development, RIKEN Center for Integrative Medical Sciences, Yokohama, Japan
e-mail: yuri.takehara@riken.jp; momozawa@riken.jp

M. Arai et al. (eds.), *Practical Guide to Hereditary Breast and Ovarian Cancer IV*,
https://doi.org/10.1007/978-981-95-6580-1_4

and surveillance of unaffected individuals [1], especially for actionable high-risk genes (more than fourfold risk relative to the population) such as *BRCA1* and *BRCA2*. Simultaneously, an increasing number of moderate-risk gene carriers (twofold to fourfold relative risk) have been identified, for which consensus on clinical management remains under discussion. Among these genes, *CHEK2* is one of the most frequently detected moderate-risk genes in multigene panel testing for patients with female breast cancer [2].

Several factors contribute to the limited clinical utility of moderate-risk genes [3–5] compared to high-risk genes, such as *BRCA1* or *BRCA2*. The American College of Medical Genetics and Genomics (ACMG) cites the complexities in establishing the cancer spectrum and penetrance for *CHEK2* heterozygotes as a major challenge [4], which stems from factors such as early studies that focused solely on a specific founder variant in Europe (e.g., c.1100delC), variation in penetrance estimates depending on study design and population, and insufficient characterization of rare missense variants.

In addition to these gene-specific challenges, it is important to consider that the associated cancer types may vary across regions depending on differences in cancer incidence [6]. This indicates the importance of region-specific evaluation of the impact of GPVs [7]. Nevertheless, most previous studies focused on European populations, and even meta-analyses included a small proportion of other populations, including Japanese [8–11]. This lack of population-specific data complicates the development of clear clinical management guidelines for carriers of *CHEK2* GPVs in non-European populations.

To address this gap and explore how to utilize the data on *CHEK2* in clinical practice, particularly in Japan, we reviewed recent reports on *CHEK2*-associated cancers and summarized the findings of our latest study investigating the association between *CHEK2* GPVs and cancer risk in Japan.

2 *CHEK2*-Associated Cancer

Cancers associated with *CHEK2* GPVs have been investigated in previous studies, reporting associations with cancer types beyond female breast cancer. However, the findings have been often inconsistent across the literature [4, 12]. To provide an overview of the current evidence base, we summarized the literature reporting hazard ratios or odds ratios that were either cited in the National Comprehensive Cancer Network (NCCN) guidelines [5, 13], the ACMG clinical resources [4], or published thereafter with a large sample size [9–11] (Table 1).

The association between *CHEK2* GPVs and colorectal cancer remains inconsistent in the literature. The association was originally suggested through the analysis of c.1100delC [14–17], while a recent large-scale association analysis showed no association between an increased risk of colorectal cancer and *CHEK2* GPVs [9, 11]. Given these data, the NCCN guidelines have been updated to state that GPVs in *CHEK2* do not increase the estimated absolute risk of colorectal cancer and that

Table 1 Other cancers associated with *CHEK2* GPVs reported in the literatures

Cancer	Literature	Study design	Analyzed variants	Study population	Risk assessment
Colorectal	Weischer et al., 2007	Prospective study Copenhagen City Heart Study participants	c.1100delC	2 colorectal cancers from 46 c.1100del heterozygotes 208 colorectal cancers from 9,171 noncarriers	Age-adjusted: OR = 1.7 (95%CI 0.4–6.7) Multi-factorially adjusted: OR = 1.6 (95%CI 0.4–6.5)
	Xiang et al., 2011 Katona et al., 2017	Meta-analysis (unselected, familial, or sporadic colorectal cancer)	c.1100delC	Unselected colorectal cancer: 54 carriers of 4,194 cases 55 carriers of 10,010 controls	Unselected colorectal cancer: OR = 2.11 (95%CI 1.41–3.16), $p = 0.0003$ Revised data: unselected colorectal cancer OR = 1.8 (95% CI: 1.2–2.7)
	Ma et al., 2014	Meta-analysis	c.1100delC, p.Ile157Thr	c.1100delC: 3,874 cases and 11,630 controls p.I157T: 6,042 cases and 17,051 controls	c.1100delC: OR = 1.88 (95%CI 1.29–2.73), $p = 0.001$ p.Ile157Thr: OR = 1.56 (95%CI 1.32–1.84), $p = 1.22 \times 10^{-7}$
	Näslund-Koch et al., 2016	Population based The Copenhagen General Population Study participants	c.1100delC heterozygous	8 colorectal cancers from 670 c.1100delC heterozygotes 1,123 colorectal cancers from 86,305 noncarriers	HR = 0.86 (95%CI 0.43–1.72), $p = 0.68$
	Bychkovsky et al., 2022	Retrospective cohort study of participants tested for cancer predisposition at Ambry Genetics	All GPVs (excluding lower risk *CHEK2* variants: p. Ile157Thr, p. Ser428Phe, and p. Thr476Met)	109 carriers of 2,684 individuals with colorectal cancer 2,015 carriers of 31,565 individuals without colorectal cancer	OR = 0.62 (95%CI 0.51–0.76), $p < 0.001$

(continued)

Table 1 (continued)

Cancer	Literature	Study design	Analyzed variants	Study population	Risk assessment
Prostate	Weischer et al., 2007	Prospective study Copenhagen City Heart Study participants	c.1100delC	2 prostate cancers from 21 c.1100delC heterozygotes 114 prostate cancers from 4,094 noncarriers	Age-adjusted: OR = 2.3 (95%CI 0.6–9.5) Multi-factorially adjusted: OR = 2.3 (95%CI 0.6–9.5)
	Wang et al., 2015	Meta-analysis	c.1100delC, c.444+1G>A, p.Ile157Thr	6,409 cases and 11,634 controls	c.1100delC: OR = 3.29 (95%CI 1.85–5.85), $p < 0.001$ c.444+1G>A: OR = 1.59 (95%CI 0.93–2.71), $p = 0.09$ p.Ile157Thr: 1.80 (95%CI 1.51–2.14), $p < 0.001$
	Näslund-Koch et al., 2016	Population-based study of the Copenhagen General Population Study participants	c.1100delC	18 prostate cancers from 289 c.1100delC heterozygotes 1,322 prostate cancers from 38,725 noncarriers	HR = 1.60 (95%CI 1.00–2.56), $p = 0.05$
	Pritchard et al., 2016	Case-control study Metastatic prostate cancer vs ExAC or primary prostate cancer (TCGA)	All GPVs (excluding p.Ile157Thr)	10 carriers of 692 metastatic prostate cancer cases 314 carriers of 53,105 controls from Exome Aggregation Consortium 2 carriers of 499 primary prostate cancer cases from the Cancer Genome Atlas cohort	Metastatic prostate cancer vs ExAC: OR = 3.1 (95%CI 1.5–5.6) $p = 0.002$ Metastatic prostate cancer vs primary prostate cancer (TCGA): OR = 4.7 (95%CI 2.2–8.5) $p = <0.001$
	Wu et al., 2018	Case-case study (Lethal versus low-risk localized prostate cancer) Individuals recruited at multiple centers in the USA or at a single center in China	c.1100delC	(European American) 8 c.1100del carriers of 624 patients with lethal prostate cancer 2 c.1100del carriers of 1223 patients with low-risk localized prostate cancers	OR (European American) = 7.86 (95%CI 1.67–37.11), $p = 0.0038$
	Ivarsdottir et al., 2024	Meta-analysis	LOF variants	21,697 cases 320,527 controls	OR = 1.88, $p = 4.40 \times 10^{-13}$
	Mitchell, et al., 2025	Meta-analysis	Flex-damaging variants[b]	158 carriers of 19,926 cases 979 carriers of 187,699 controls	OR = 1.69 (95% CI 1.41–2.01), $p = 2.69 \times 10^{-8}$

Renal	Weischer et al., 2007	Prospective study of Copenhagen City Heart Study participants	c.1100delC	3 renal cancers from 46 c.1100delC heterozygotes 30 renal cancers from 9,183 noncarriers	Age-adjusted: OR = 10.8 (95%CI 2.6–45.7) Multi-factorially adjusted: OR = 9.8 (95%CI 2.3–41.2)
	Näslund-Koch et al., 2016	Population-based study of the Copenhagen General Population Study participants	c.1100delC	4 renal cancers from 670 c.1100delC heterozygotes 134 renal cancers from 86,304 noncarriers	HR = 3.61 (95%CI 1.33–9.79), $p = 0.01$
	Carlo et al., 2018	Retrospective multicenter cohort study (advanced RCC cases [stage III-IV] in USA)	All GPVs	254 patients with advanced renal cell carcinoma Non-cancer cohort from ExAC	OR = 3.0 (95%CI 1.3–5.8), $p = 0.003$
	Bychkovsky et al., 2022	Retrospective cohort study of participants tested for cancer predisposition at Ambry Genetics	All GPVs (excluding lower risk *CHEK2* variants: p. Ile157Thr, p. Ser428Phe, and p. Thr476Met)	36 carriers of 250 individuals with renal cancer 2,088 carriers of 33,984 individuals without renal cancer	OR = 2.57 (95%CI 1.75–3.68), $p < 0.001$
	Ivarsdottir, et al., 2024	Meta-analysis	LOF + deleterious missense variants[c]	4,627 cases 851,840 controls	OR = 1.67, $p = 1.10 \times 10^{-6}$
Thyroid	Näslund-Koch et al., 2016	Population-based study of the Copenhagen General Population Study participants	c.1100delC	5 thyroid cancers from 670 c.1100delC heterozygotes 99 thyroid cancers from 86,303 noncarriers	HR = 1.27 (95%CI 0.18–9.09), $p = 0.81$
	Bychkovsky et al., 2022	Retrospective cohort study of participants tested for cancer predisposition at Ambry Genetics	All GPVs (excluding lower risk *CHEK2* variants: p. Ile157Thr, p. Ser428Phe, and p. Thr476Met)	74 carriers of 770 individuals with thyroid cancer 2,050 carriers of 33,466 individuals without thyroid cancer	OR = 1.63 (95%CI 1.26–2.08), $p < 0.001$
	Ivarsdottir, et al., 2024	Meta-analysis	LOF + deleterious missense variants[c]	2,366 cases 788,307 controls	OR = 2.25, $p = 4.40 \times 10^{-10}$

Abbreviation: *GPVs* germline pathogenic variants, *LOF* loss of function

[a]The listed studies were either cited in the National Comprehensive Cancer Network guidelines or the clinical practice resource of the American College of Medical Genetics and Genomics, or were published subsequently with large sample sizes

[b]Variants included met the following criteria: gnomAD minor allele frequency (MAF) ≤0.05%, gnomAD popmax MAF ≤0.1%, internal MAF ≤0.1%, maximum number of QC-failed samples ≤4, and REVEL score ≥0.25

[c]Moderate impact indels and predicted deleterious missense variants with MAF <2%, if considered predicted deleterious by at least one of the following prediction methods: (1) MetaSVM; (2) MetaLR using variants available in dbNSFP v4.1c; or (3) CADD score ≥25

general population screening is appropriate if probands do not have a personal or first-degree family history [13].

An association between prostate cancer and *CHEK2* GPVs has also been reported, which is described with "emerging evidence" in the NCCN guidelines. The association was initially indicated through the analysis of c.1100delC [16–18] in specific categories, such as metastatic or aggressive prostate cancer [18, 19], but recent large-scale studies have shown a significant association irrespective of cancer status [10, 11].

Several studies have shown that thyroid and renal cancers are associated with *CHEK2* GPVs [9, 11, 16, 17, 20]. Early studies focused on specific variants (i.e., c.1100delC) or specific statuses (i.e., high-stage) and had limited sample sizes [16, 17, 20]. Recently, some larger-scale studies have reported associations between *CHEK2* GPVs, or other deleterious variants, and moderately increased cancer risks [9, 11]. However, both the NCCN and the ACMG state that the data regarding increased risks for these two cancers are inconclusive.

Taken together, these findings have led the NCCN guidelines and the ACMG clinical resources to discuss potential associations with specific cancers, including colorectal, prostate, renal, and thyroid cancers, though the evidence remains controversial or limited [4, 13]. This lack of consistency has obstructed the development of clinical management strategies for *CHEK2* GPV carriers, in contrast to the well-established approaches for *BRCA1/2* GPV carriers, even in the European population [4]. For breast cancer, a previous study reported that additional MRI screening could be beneficial for *CHEK2* carriers regardless of individual risk profiles [21]. However, evidence supporting additional systematic clinical intervention for *CHEK2* GPV carriers before cancer onset remains limited. Furthermore, regarding prostate cancer, due to insufficient evidence on appropriate surveillance of *CHEK2* GPV carriers, this issue has been addressed based on evidence from studies developed for *BRCA2* GPV carriers [4].

3 Large-Scale Case-Control Study for *CHEK2* in Japan

Although region-specific data are essential for translating research data into clinical practice for genetic medicine, there is limited evidence on the clinical relevance of *CHEK2* GPVs in Japan. To address this, we recently reported that a large-scale unselected case-control analysis of 23 cancer types using 112,141 DNA samples from Biobank Japan [22], which is a multi-centered hospital-based registry across Japan [23–25]. In this study, we incorporated the functional analysis of missense variants using established assays [26] and defined functionally impaired variants as GPVs as well as pathogenic or likely pathogenic variants in ClinVar, and predicted loss-of-function variants. Among 77 GPVs, including 36 functionally impaired missense variants, we observed a founder variant, p.Arg521Trp, specific to the Japanese population, through functional analysis. Association analysis revealed that *CHEK2* GPVs were significantly associated with female breast cancer (OR, 1.8 [95% CI, 1.3–2.6], $P = 1.2 \times 10^{-3}$) and prostate cancer (OR, 1.8 [1.2–2.6] $P = 1.7 \times 10^{-3}$) in the population. Regarding clinical characteristics, we observed no significant differences between *CHEK2* GPVs carriers and non-carriers in terms of age at diagnosis, pathological features (proportion of triple-negative breast cancer and prostate cancer with a Gleason score of 8–10), or overall survival. These findings suggested that the expected benefits of additional systematic clinical management of *CHEK2* GPV carriers may be limited.

4 Conclusion

To apply the findings on *CHEK2*, a moderate-risk gene, in clinical practice, region-specific data on its association with cancer types are important. Our study identified a founder variant specific to the Japanese population and demonstrated a concordance between the spectrum of *CHEK2*-associated cancers in Japan and those previously reported in European populations. These findings provide important insights that may support clinical decision-making regarding the medical management of *CHEK2* carriers. Further accumulation of clinical data is warranted to determine the most appropriate interventions for these individuals.

References

1. Samadder NJ, Riegert-Johnson D, Boardman L, Rhodes D, Wick M, Okuno S, et al. Comparison of universal genetic testing vs guideline-directed targeted testing for patients with hereditary cancer syndrome. JAMA Oncol. 2021;7(2):230–7.
2. Dorling L, Carvalho S, Allen J, González-Neira A, Luccarini C, Wahlström C, et al. Breast cancer risk genes – association analysis in more than 113,000 women. N Engl J Med. 2021;384(5):428–39.
3. Bedrosian I, Somerfield MR, Achatz MI, Boughey JC, Curigliano G, Friedman S, et al. Germline testing in patients with breast cancer: ASCO-Society of Surgical Oncology guideline. J Clin Oncol. 2024;42(5):584–604.
4. Hanson H, Astiazaran-Symonds E, Amendola LM, Balmaña J, Foulkes WD, James P, et al. Management of individuals with germline pathogenic/likely pathogenic variants in CHEK2: a clinical practice resource of the American College of Medical Genetics and Genomics (ACMG). Genet Med. 2023;25(10):100870.
5. National Comprehensive Cancer Network (NCCN). Genetic/familial high-risk assessment: breast, ovarian, pancreatic, and prostate. Version 3.2025. Accessed 7 July 2025.
6. Momozawa Y, Sasai R, Usui Y, Shiraishi K, Iwasaki Y, Taniyama Y, et al. Expansion of cancer risk profile for BRCA1 and BRCA2 pathogenic variants. JAMA Oncol. 2022;8(6):871–8.
7. Usui Y, Momozawa Y. Personalized medicine with germline pathogenic variants: importance of population- and region-wide evidence. Cancer Sci. 2023;114(10):3816–24.
8. Stern RH. Correspondence on "Management of individuals with germline pathogenic/likely pathogenic variants in CHEK2: A clinical practice resource of the American College of Medical Genetics and Genomics (ACMG)" by Hanson et al. Genet Med. 2023:101031.
9. Bychkovsky BL, Agaoglu NB, Horton C, Zhou J, Yussuf A, Hemyari P, et al. Differences in cancer phenotypes among frequent CHEK2 variants and implications for clinical care-checking CHEK2. JAMA Oncol. 2022;8(11):1598–606.

10. Mitchell J, Camacho N, Shea P, Stopsack KH, Joseph V, Burren OS, et al. Assessing the contribution of rare protein-coding germline variants to prostate cancer risk and severity in 37,184 cases. Nat Commun. 2025;16(1):1779.
11. Ivarsdottir EV, Gudmundsson J, Tragante V, Sveinbjornsson G, Kristmundsdottir S, Stacey SN, et al. Gene-based burden tests of rare germline variants identify six cancer susceptibility genes. Nat Genet. 2024;56(11):2422–33.
12. Stolarova L, Kleiblova P, Janatova M, Soukupova J, Zemankova P, Macurek L, et al. Germline variants in cancer predisposition: stalemate rather than checkmate. Cells. 2020;9(12):2675.
13. National Comprehensive Cancer Network (NCCN). Genetic/familial high-risk assessment: colorectal, endometrial, and gastric. Version 1.2025. Accessed 7 July 2025.
14. Ma X, Zhang B, Zheng W. Genetic variants associated with colorectal cancer risk: comprehensive research synopsis, meta-analysis, and epidemiological evidence. Gut. 2014;63(2):326–36.
15. Xiang HP, Geng XP, Ge WW, Li H. Meta-analysis of CHEK2 1100delC variant and colorectal cancer susceptibility. Eur J Cancer. 2011;47(17):2546–51.
16. Näslund-Koch C, Nordestgaard BG, Bojesen SE. Increased risk for other cancers in addition to breast cancer for CHEK2*1100delC heterozygotes estimated from the Copenhagen general population study. J Clin Oncol. 2016;34(11):1208–16.
17. Weischer M, Bojesen SE, Tybjaerg-Hansen A, Axelsson CK, Nordestgaard BG. Increased risk of breast cancer associated with CHEK2*1100delC. J Clin Oncol. 2007;25(1):57–63.
18. Wu Y, Yu H, Zheng SL, Na R, Mamawala M, Landis T, et al. A comprehensive evaluation of CHEK2 germline mutations in men with prostate cancer. Prostate. 2018;78(8):607–15.
19. Pritchard CC, Mateo J, Walsh MF, De Sarkar N, Abida W, Beltran H, et al. Inherited DNA-repair gene mutations in men with metastatic prostate cancer. N Engl J Med. 2016;375(5):443–53.
20. Carlo MI, Mukherjee S, Mandelker D, Vijai J, Kemel Y, Zhang L, et al. Prevalence of germline mutations in cancer susceptibility genes in patients with advanced renal cell carcinoma. JAMA Oncol. 2018;4(9):1228–35.
21. Lowry KP, Geuzinge HA, Stout NK, Alagoz O, Hampton J, Kerlikowske K, et al. Breast cancer screening strategies for women with ATM, CHEK2, and PALB2 pathogenic variants: a comparative modeling analysis. JAMA Oncol. 2022;8(4):587–96.
22. Takehara Y, Usui Y, Stolarova L, Kleiblova P, Iwasaki Y, Johnson TA, et al. Case-Control Study for 23 Cancer Types With Functional Analysis of CHEK2: Risk Estimation and Clinical Recommendations in East Asia. JCO Precis Oncol. 2025;9:e2400945
23. Hirata M, Kamatani Y, Nagai A, Kiyohara Y, Ninomiya T, Tamakoshi A, et al. Cross-sectional analysis of BioBank Japan clinical data: a large cohort of 200,000 patients with 47 common diseases. J Epidemiol. 2017;27(3S):S9–S21.
24. Nagai A, Hirata M, Kamatani Y, Muto K, Matsuda K, Kiyohara Y, et al. Overview of the BioBank Japan Project: study design and profile. J Epidemiol. 2017;27(3S):S2–8.
25. Hirata M, Nagai A, Kamatani Y, Ninomiya T, Tamakoshi A, Yamagata Z, et al. Overview of BioBank Japan follow-up data in 32 diseases. J Epidemiol. 2017;27(3S):S22–S8.
26. Stolarova L, Kleiblova P, Zemankova P, Stastna B, Janatova M, Soukupova J, et al. ENIGMA CHEK2gether Project: a comprehensive study identifies functionally impaired CHEK2 germline missense variants associated with increased breast cancer risk. Clin Cancer Res. 2023;29(16):3037–50.

Large-Scale Functional Analysis and Evaluation of Pathogenicity in *BRCA2*

Tatsuki Yamazoe and Yukihide Momozawa

Abstract Germline pathogenic variants of *BRCA2* are significantly associated with a high risk of several cancers. Although genetic testing allows for individual risk management, the large number of variants of uncertain significance (VUSs) identified through genetic testing poses a significant challenge to clinical utility. Owing to insufficient clinical evidence to determine the pathogenicity of these variants, various in vitro assays must be developed. Various functional evaluations have been performed using assays based on the different functions of *BRCA2*. These data were considered as strong evidence for interpreting the pathogenicity of VUSs. The accumulation of functional data from these assays has enabled significant progress in addressing the VUSs. However, several issues remain regarding the clinical application of functional annotations. Here, we summarize several functional assays for the reclassification of VUSs and the contribution of functionally abnormal variants to cancer risk. Subsequently, we discuss the challenges in the clinical utility of functional data and future studies that could overcome these challenges.

Keywords BRCA2 · Variant of uncertain significance · Cancer genetics

1 Introduction

BRCA2 encodes a large protein that plays a crucial role in maintaining genomic integrity, and germline pathogenic variants of this gene significantly increase the risk of several cancer types [1–3]. The identification of pathogenic variants allows for individual risk management, such as surveillance, prophylactic surgery, and targeted therapies. However, genetic testing often reveals variants of uncertain significance (VUSs) based on the American College of Medical Genetics and Genomics

---

T. Yamazoe · Y. Momozawa (✉)
Laboratory for Genotyping Development, RIKEN Center for Integrative Medical Sciences, Yokohama, Japan
e-mail: tatsuki.yamazoe@riken.jp; momozawa@riken.jp

M. Arai et al. (eds.), *Practical Guide to Hereditary Breast and Ovarian Cancer IV*,
https://doi.org/10.1007/978-981-95-6580-1_5

and Association for Molecular Pathogenicity (ACMG/AMP) guidelines [4]. Additional functional analyses are required to interpret the pathogenicity of VUSs. Here, we introduce various reported functional studies for the reclassification of VUSs in *BRCA2* to highlight the importance of accumulating these functional data. We then discuss the challenges involved in applying these functional data to clinical practice.

2 In Vitro Functional Analysis for *BRCA2* Variant Classification

Table 1 shows the characteristics of various functional analyses used for the reclassification of VUSs. Homology-directed repair (HDR) is a key function of *BRCA2*, and HDR deficiency contributes to cancer development [5]. A DR-GFP reporter assay was designed to assess the HDR activity by measuring the repair of I-SceI-induced DSB through GFP expression. This reporter was used to evaluate the pathogenicity of 462 variants in the DNA-binding domain (DBD) by assessing HDR deficiency complementation through the expression of full-length human *BRCA2* cDNA in *BRCA2*-deficient V-C8 hamster lung fibroblasts [6]. This study showed high sensitivity and specificity based on a set of 21 known pathogenic and 35 known benign missense variants. When the functional annotation of 442 variants (excluding known abnormal splicing variants and functionally intermediate variants) was incorporated into the ACMG/AMP framework, 326 variants were successfully classified.

This reporter assay was also used in a *BRCA2*-deficient human colorectal carcinoma cell line [7]. The HDR activities of 108 VUSs that were not included in the ClinVar database were analyzed in this study. Based on the ACMG/AMP framework using these functional data and their unique integrated in silico prediction models, 101 VUSs were successfully reclassified.

MANO-B methods were developed for the high-throughput functional evaluation of VUSs using *BRCA2*-deficient DLD-1 cells stably expressing *BRCA2* variants [8]. Using this method, the pathogenicity of 244 missense variants, including 186 VUSs, was evaluated by measuring their sensitivity to polyadenosine diphosphate-ribose polymerase inhibitors in a mixed population of cells harboring the individual variants. This method showed a strong correlation with the International Agency for Research on Cancer classification. Of the 186 VUSs, 126 were functionally classified as normal, 23 as intermediate, and 37 as abnormal.

Two recently published papers described the application of a high-throughput assay called multiplexed assays of variant effects (MAVEs) for the functional evaluation of *BRCA2* variants [9, 10]. These studies introduced all possible single-nucleotide variants (SNVs) into the endogenous *BRCA2* gene using CRISPR/Cas9 knock-in-based saturation genome editing, enabling a comprehensive functional evaluation that includes the effect of variants on mRNA splicing. Both studies

Table 1 In vitro functional assays for the clinical interpretation of BRCA2 variants

Study	Assay	Cell line	Phenotype	Variant library	N of variants	Sensitivity (95%CI)	Specificity (95% CI)	Limitation
Huang et al. 2025	MAVE	Human haploid HAP1 cell	Cell growth	Endogenous locus	6959	99% (97–100%)	99% (97–100%)	Dominant-negative variants cannot be evaluated No functional data in regions outside the DBD
Sahu et al. 2025	MAVE	Humanized mouse ES cell	Sensitivity to PARP inhibitor	Endogenous locus	6551	88% (84–92%)	86% (83–89%)	Dominant-negative variants cannot be evaluated No functional data in regions outside the DBD Physiological differences may affect functional evaluation

(continued)

Table 1 (continued)

Study	Assay	Cell line	Phenotype	Variant library	N of variants	Sensitivity (95%CI)	Specificity (95% CI)	Limitation
Hu et al. 2024	HDR assay	Hamster lung fibroblast V-C8 cell	GFP reporter	Transient expression	462	100% (79–100%)	100% (93–100%)	Splicing-altering variants cannot be evaluated No functional data in regions outside the DBD Variants that are not involved in HDR phenotypes cannot be evaluated Physiological differences may affect functional evaluation
Guo et al. 2023	HR assay	Human colorectal adenocarcinoma DLD-1 cell	GFP reporter	Transient expression	108	–	–	Splicing-altering variants cannot be evaluated Variants that are not involved in HDR phenotypes cannot be evaluated

Ikegami et al. 2020	MANO-B	Human colorectal adenocarcinoma DLD-1 cell	Sensitivity to PARP inhibitor	Exogenous expression	244	95% (77–100%)[a]	95% (82–99%)[a]	Splicing-altering variants cannot be evaluated Variants that are not involved in HDR phenotypes cannot be evaluated

[a]The sensitivity and specificity were calculated using the data for 0.5 μM niraparib

analyzed more than 95% of the possible SNVs in DBD and demonstrated high sensitivity and specificity when validated using known pathogenic and benign variants reported in ClinVar. By incorporating MAVE functional data into the ACMG/AMP framework, 6351 and 5819 SNVs were classified in MAVE studies using HAP1 and mouse embryonic stem cell lines, respectively.

3 Clinical Relevance in *BRCA2*-Related Cancer

Some studies have performed association analyses between pooled functionally abnormal variants and breast and ovarian cancers [6, 10] (Table 2). Both functionally abnormal HDR variants and MAVE pathogenic variants were significantly associated with a high risk (odds ratio (OR) >4.0) of breast and ovarian cancers. These functionally abnormal variants showed attenuated OR compared to protein-truncating variants, indicating that many missense pathogenic variants have only a weak or partial effect on *BRCA2* function and a moderate risk of cancer compared to protein-truncating variants.

Although *BRCA2* pathogenic variants are associated with various types of cancer, breast cancer is typically used to evaluate the clinical relevance of functionally abnormal variants. Variants in certain regions affect the risk of developing different types of cancer. For example, *BRCA2* has three breast cancer cluster regions and two ovarian cancer cluster regions that are associated with a relatively high risk of breast and ovarian cancers, respectively [11]. Similar regions have been reported for pancreatic [12] and prostate [13] cancers. A better understanding of the contribution of these functionally abnormal variants to *BRCA2*-related cancers can provide beneficial information for the clinical application of functional evaluations.

Table 2 Associations of functionally abnormal variants with the risk of breast and ovarian cancers

	Case		Control		Cancer risk	
	No. of variants	No. tested	No. of variants	No. tested	OR (95% CI)	*P* value
Breast cancer in HAP1-based MAVE study[a]						
MAVE missense Pathogenic category	261	197,659	60	181,964	4.34 (3.27–5.85)	4.35×10^{-22}
ACMG missense Pathogenic/Likely pathogenic	210	197,659	29	181,964	6.96 (4.77–10.56)	5.87×10^{-21}
PTV in DBD	469	197,659	63	181,964	6.68 (5.19–8.74)	1.91×10^{-44}
Ovarian cancer in HAP1-based MAVE study[a]						
MAVE missense Pathogenic category	57	24,981	60	181,964	7.76 (5.34–11.29)	1.39×10^{-25}
ACMG missense Pathogenic/Likely pathogenic	43	24,981	29	181,964	11.69 (7.27–19.17)	2.28×10^{-22}
PTV in DBD	85	24,981	63	181,964	9.35 (6.79–12.93)	1.51×10^{-40}
Breast cancer in V-C8-based HDR assay[b]						
Functionally abnormal missense (HDR <1.49)	104	82,372	30	123,464	5.2 (3.47–7.9)	9.99×10^{-19}
ACMG missense Pathogenic/Likely pathogenic	103	82,372	30	123,464	5.15 (3.43–7.83)	1.88×10^{-18}
PTV in DBD	211	82,372	37	123,464	8.56 (6.03–12.36)	1.37×10^{-48}
Ovarian cancer in V-C8-based HDR assay[b]						
Functionally abnormal missense (HDR <1.49)	24	10,960	30	123,464	9.02 (5.15–15.84)	9.02×10^{-13}
ACMG missense Pathogenic/Likely pathogenic	23	10,960	30	123,464	8.64 (4.85–15.33)	4.95×10^{-12}
PTV in DBD	41	10,960	37	123,464	12.5 (7.92–19.66)	2.58×10^{-24}

[a]Cases: patients with breast cancer and from patients with ovarian cancer (all had cancer genetic testing by Ambry Genetics); Controls: gnomAD v.4 (women), excluding the UK Biobank
[b]Cases: patients with breast cancer and from patients with ovarian cancer (all had cancer genetic testing by Ambry Genetics); Controls: gnomAD 2.1 and 3.1 non-cancer females and CARRIERS population-based controls

4 Conclusion

VUS issues in clinical practice have become less significant because of the accumulation of functional evaluations from various assays. MAVE is a particularly time- and cost-effective experiment that is expected to significantly improve the clinical annotation of VUSs [14]. However, many functional studies have not evaluated the pathogenicity of *BRCA2* variants in regions outside the DBD, as only a limited number of variants have been established as benchmarks in these regions. Furthermore, the clinical relevance of functionally abnormal variants in *BRCA2*-related cancers, other than breast and ovarian cancers, has not been evaluated. These issues could be overcome in future studies evaluating the clinical relevance of functional analyses using large case-control datasets covering all *BRCA2*-related cancers.

References

1. Wooster R, Bignell G, Lancaster J, et al. Identification of the breast cancer susceptibility gene BRCA2. Nature. 1995;378:789–92. https://doi.org/10.1038/378789a0.
2. Hu C, Hart SN, Polley EC, et al. Association between inherited germline mutations in cancer predisposition genes and risk of pancreatic cancer. JAMA. 2018;319:2401–9. https://doi.org/10.1001/jama.2018.6228.
3. Oh M, Alkhushaym N, Fallatah S, et al. The association of BRCA1 and BRCA2 mutations with prostate cancer risk, frequency, and mortality: a meta-analysis. Prostate. 2019;79:880–95. https://doi.org/10.1002/pros.23795.
4. Parsons MT, de la Hoya M, Richardson ME, et al. Evidence-based recommendations for gene-specific ACMG/AMP variant classification from the ClinGen ENIGMA BRCA1 and BRCA2 Variant Curation Expert Panel. Am J Hum Genet. 2024;111:2044–58. https://doi.org/10.1016/j.ajhg.2024.07.013.
5. Creeden JF, Nanavaty NS, Einloth KR, et al. Homologous recombination proficiency in ovarian and breast cancer patients. BMC Cancer. 2021;21:1154. https://doi.org/10.1186/s12885-021-08863-9.
6. Hu C, Huang H, Na J, et al. Functional analysis and clinical classification of 462 germline BRCA2 missense variants affecting the DNA binding domain. Am J Hum Genet. 2024. https://doi.org/10.1016/j.ajhg.2024.02.002.
7. Guo Q, Ji S, Takeuchi K, et al. Functional evaluation of BRCA1/2 variants of unknown significance with homologous recombination assay and integrative in silico prediction model. J Hum Genet. 2023;68:849–57. https://doi.org/10.1038/s10038-023-01194-6.
8. Ikegami M, Kohsaka S, Ueno T, et al. High-throughput functional evaluation of BRCA2 variants of unknown significance. Nat Commun. 2020;11:2573. https://doi.org/10.1038/s41467-020-16141-8.
9. Sahu S, Galloux M, Southon E, et al. Saturation genome editing-based clinical classification of BRCA2 variants. Nature. 2025:1–8. https://doi.org/10.1038/s41586-024-08349-1.
10. Huang H, Hu C, Na J, et al. Functional evaluation and clinical classification of BRCA2 variants. Nature. 2025;638:528–37. https://doi.org/10.1038/s41586-024-08388-8.
11. Rebbeck TR, Mitra N, Wan F, et al. Association of type and location of BRCA1 and BRCA2 mutations with risk of breast and ovarian cancer. JAMA. 2015;313:1347–61. https://doi.org/10.1001/jama.2014.5985.

12. Chian JS, Xu W, Wang SM. Pancreatic cancer cluster region identified in BRCA2. J Med Genet. 2023;60:1052–6. https://doi.org/10.1136/jmg-2022-109111.
13. Nyberg T, Frost D, Barrowdale D, et al. Prostate cancer risk by *BRCA2* genomic regions. Eur Urol. 2020;78:494–7. https://doi.org/10.1016/j.eururo.2020.05.005.
14. McEwen AE, Tejura M, Fayer S, et al. Multiplexed assays of variant effect for clinical variant interpretation. Nat Rev Genet. 2025:1–18. https://doi.org/10.1038/s41576-025-00870-x.

Integrating *BRCA1* and *BRCA2* Pathogenic Variants with Polygenic Risk Scores

Ryoko Yamada and Yukihide Momozawa

Abstract Germline pathogenic variants of *BRCA1* and *BRCA2* confer substantially elevated lifetime risks of breast, ovarian, prostate, and other cancers, although they occur at low frequencies in the population. In contrast, common single-nucleotide polymorphisms (SNPs) individually exert only small effects but are widespread in the population. When aggregated as polygenic risk scores (PRSs), these common variants play a complementary role in enhancing risk prediction, particularly when integrated with rare high-penetrance variants to enable more accurate and nuanced risk stratification. Previous large-scale analyses have demonstrated that the PRSs further stratify the risk among *BRCA1* and *BRCA2* carriers, and the PRSs have been incorporated into clinical risk assessment tools for female breast cancer. However, its limitations include restricted validation across non-European populations and its applicability to only a few cancer types. To address these gaps, we integrated *BRCA1* and *BRCA2* carrier status with PRSs in East Asian populations using BioBank Japan data. The preliminary results suggested heterogeneous contributions of PRSs by cancer type. This integrative approach holds promise for precise prevention and individualized surveillance strategies.

Keywords Genome · Large-scale analysis · Polygenic risk scores · Risk prediction

1 Introduction

Genetic factors are fundamental determinants of cancer susceptibility and individual risks. Germline pathogenic variants of *BRCA1* and *BRCA2* are among the most well-established genetic risk factors for various cancers, including breast, ovarian,

R. Yamada · Y. Momozawa (✉)
Laboratory for Genotyping Development, RIKEN Center for Integrative Medical Sciences, Yokohama, Japan
e-mail: ryoko.yamada@a.riken.jp; momozawa@riken.jp

M. Arai et al. (eds.), *Practical Guide to Hereditary Breast and Ovarian Cancer IV*,
https://doi.org/10.1007/978-981-95-6580-1_6

pancreatic, and prostate cancers. Carriers of these variants face a markedly elevated lifetime risk, with relative risk estimates often exceeding five- to tenfold compared to that of the general population [1]. However, these rare variants occur at low frequencies in the general population, limiting their contribution to the overall disease burden. Conversely, common germline variants, most often single-nucleotide polymorphisms (SNPs), are individually associated with small increases in risk but occur at high frequencies, indicating that their cumulative impact on disease prevalence may be considerable [2]. Over the past few decades, genome-wide association studies have identified numerous such loci associated with cancer susceptibility [3–5]. Thus, both rare high-penetrance and common low-risk variants are essential components of genetic susceptibility to cancer.

Polygenic risk scores (PRSs) aggregate the effects of common variants into a single quantitative measure for each individual. The construction of a PRS involves identifying disease-associated SNPs, applying rigorous quality control and linkage disequilibrium pruning, and calculating the weighted allele sum [6]. PRSs are standardized relative to a reference population, allowing percentile-based risk stratification; individuals in the highest percentile may have several-fold elevated risk compared to those in the lowest percentile. Thus, PRSs have emerged as a promising tool for refining genetic risk predictions [7].

2 Clinical Implications of PRSs in Oncology

The integration of *BRCA1* and *BRCA2* carrier status with PRSs offers opportunities to enhance risk stratification and inform personalized surveillance and preventive strategies. Large-scale analyses conducted by the Consortium of Investigators of Modifiers of *BRCA1* and *BRCA2* (CIMBA) have demonstrated that PRSs can effectively stratify cancer risk, even among individuals carrying pathogenic variants of *BRCA1* or *BRCA2*. For instance, *BRCA1* carriers in the highest decile of the estrogen receptor (ER)-negative breast cancer PRSs exhibit a higher risk than those in the lowest decile. Specifically, among *BRCA1* carriers, the predicted breast cancer risk at the 10th percentile of the PRSs was 21% by age 50 and 56% by age 80, whereas at the 90th percentile, the corresponding risks increased to 39% and 75%, respectively [8]. In female breast cancer, the PRSs have already been incorporated into the clinical risk assessment tool CanRisk, which integrates genetic, lifestyle, and hormonal factors to provide individualized risk estimates [9]. This integration underscores the potential clinical utility of the PRSs as an important determinant of cancer susceptibility.

However, a major limitation is that most PRSs models have been developed and validated primarily in European populations, raising concerns regarding their transferability and predictive accuracy in diverse ancestral groups. Another limitation is that the applicability of the PRSs remains restricted to a limited range of cancer types. The PRSs have been shown to stratify the risk of ovarian and prostate cancers among *BRCA1* and *BRCA2* carriers [8, 10, 11]. Nevertheless, outside of female breast cancer, PRS-based risk prediction remains in the early stages of clinical evaluation.

3 Ongoing Research in Our Team

To explore the potential utility of integrating *BRCA1* and *BRCA2* carrier status with the PRSs in an East Asian context, we analyzed data from a large Japanese biobank, BioBank Japan. In East Asian populations, germline pathogenic variants of *BRCA1* or *BRCA2* are known to increase the risk of biliary tract, esophageal, and gastric cancers, in addition to breast, ovarian, prostate, and pancreatic cancers [12]. By combining *BRCA1* and *BRCA2* carrier status with the PRSs, this study aimed to identify subgroups at particularly elevated risk, both among *BRCA1* or *BRCA2* carriers (e.g., carriers with high PRSs who are at especially high risk) and *BRCA1* or *BRCA2* non-carriers (e.g., individuals without *BRCA1* or *BRCA2* germline pathogenic variants but with high PRSs who may reach risk levels comparable to those of carriers) (Fig. 1).

Our preliminary research, presented at the Annual Meeting of the Japanese Organization of Hereditary Breast and Ovarian Cancer 2024, suggests that the added value of PRSs integration depends strongly on the cancer type. We analyzed 12,194 prostate cancer, 11,742 female breast cancer, and 10,888 gastric cancer cases, and 69,316 non-cancer controls with imputed genotype data and sequencing data of *BRCA1* and *BRCA2*. The samples were divided into two groups: a genome-wide association study, derivation, and cross-validation of PRSs was conducted in one group, and risk estimation by integrating *BRCA1* and *BRCA2* and PRSs was performed in the other group. The results of *BRCA1*, *BRCA2*, and PRS-integrated risk estimation showed different trends according to the cancer type. In prostate cancer, when non-carriers of pathogenic variants of *BRCA1* and *BRCA2* with middle PRSs were set as a reference, non-carriers with high PRSs showed a higher risk (odds ratio [OR]: ~6.8) than carriers with low PRSs (OR: ~2.8). In breast cancer, carriers

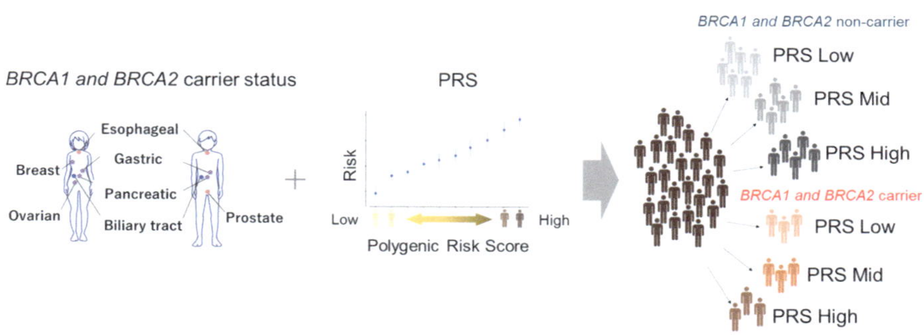

Fig. 1 Conceptual diagram of our study. Risk stratification is achieved by integrating *BRCA1* and *BRCA2* carrier status with the PRSs

of *BRCA1* and *BRCA2* showed a higher risk than non-carriers, regardless of the PRSs (OR: 10). In gastric cancer, carriers of *BRCA1* and *BRCA2* showed a higher risk than non-carriers, regardless of the PRSs, but not as high as that in breast cancer (OR: ~2). Our results suggest that the importance of integrating *BRCA1*, *BRCA2*, and PRSs for risk estimation differs according to the cancer type; evaluating PRSs in addition to *BRCA1* and *BRCA2* may help identify individuals at high risk of prostate cancer, whereas the clinical significance of integrating these factors may be limited in other cancers.

4 Conclusion

Integrating *BRCA1* and *BRCA2* pathogenic variants with the PRSs may refine cancer risk prediction by capturing both rare high-penetrance and common low-risk variants. Although the contribution of PRSs varies by cancer type and remains limited in some contexts, population- and cancer-specific models may offer the potential to advance precise prevention and individualized surveillance strategies.

Competing Interests The authors declare no conflicts of interest.

References

1. Antoniou A, et al. Average risks of breast and ovarian cancer associated with BRCA1 or BRCA2 mutations detected in case series unselected for family history: a combined analysis of 22 studies. Am J Hum Genet. 2003;72(5):1117–30.
2. Turnbull C, Sud A, Houlston RS. Cancer genetics, precision prevention and a call to action. Nat Genet. 2018;50(9):1212–8.
3. Michailidou K, et al. Association analysis identifies 65 new breast cancer risk loci. Nature. 2017;551(7678):92–4.
4. Schumacher FR, et al. Association analyses of more than 140,000 men identify 63 new prostate cancer susceptibility loci. Nat Genet. 2018;50(7):928–36.
5. Phelan CM, et al. Identification of 12 new susceptibility loci for different histotypes of epithelial ovarian cancer. Nat Genet. 2017;49(5):680–91.
6. Choi SW, Mak TS, O'Reilly PF. Tutorial: a guide to performing polygenic risk score analyses. Nat Protoc. 2020;15(9):2759–72.
7. Khera AV, et al. Genome-wide polygenic scores for common diseases identify individuals with risk equivalent to monogenic mutations. Nat Genet. 2018;50:1219–24.
8. Kuchenbaecker KB, et al. Evaluation of polygenic risk scores for breast and ovarian cancer risk prediction in BRCA1 and BRCA2 mutation carriers. J Natl Cancer Inst. 2017;109(7):djw302.
9. Lee A, et al. BOADICEA: a comprehensive breast cancer risk prediction model incorporating genetic and nongenetic risk factors. Genet Med. 2019;21(8):1708–18.
10. Barnes DR, et al. Polygenic risk scores and breast and epithelial ovarian cancer risks for carriers of BRCA1 and BRCA2 pathogenic variants. Genet Med. 2020;22(10):1653–66.

11. Barnes DR, et al. Breast and prostate cancer risks for male BRCA1 and BRCA2 pathogenic variant carriers using polygenic risk scores. J Natl Cancer Inst. 2022;114(1):109–22.
12. Momozawa Y, et al. Expansion of cancer risk profile for BRCA1 and BRCA2 pathogenic variants. JAMA Oncol. 2022;8(6):871–8.

Advances in Breast Cancer

Supporting Strategies for HBOC Unaffected Carriers

Misato Suzuki

Abstract *Background*: Hereditary breast and ovarian cancer (HBOC) syndrome, caused by germline pathogenic variants in BRCA1/2, substantially increases cancer risk (Miki et al, Science 266(5182):66–71, 1994; Wooster et al, Nature 378(6559):789–792, 1995). In Japan, unaffected carriers now have access to surveillance and risk-reducing options, still uncovered by national insurance (Daly et al, J Natl Compr Canc Netw 20(1):38–69, 2022; The Japanese Association of Medical Sciences, Guidelines for genetic testing and diagnosis in medical care [in Japanese], 2011; Ministry of Health, Labour and Welfare, Notification on insurance coverage for BRCA1/2 testing and risk-reducing surgery [in Japanese], 2020). However, long-term adherence and life-stage-sensitive support remain challenges. *Methods*: We reviewed clinical practice at St. Luke's International Hospital, focusing on institutional frameworks, evolution of genetic counseling practices, integration with oncology services, and the development of a dedicated HBOC clinic. Data from 2023 on genetic testing, surgical uptake, and clinic attendance were summarized. *Results*: In 2023, 475 genetic tests were performed, and 26 risk-reducing surgeries (16 RRM, 10 RRSO) were completed. Detailed breakdowns are shown in Table 1. Based on cumulative institutional data up to 2023, occult cancer was detected in 9 of 153 risk-reducing mastectomy (RRM) cases (5.9%) and in 4 of 198 risk-reducing salpingo-oophorectomy (RRSO) cases (2.0%). A dedicated HBOC clinic, established in January 2023, provided 395 cumulative visits within the first year, offering coordinated same-day consultations with breast surgeons, gynecologists, and genetic counselors. Counseling practices shifted toward video-based pre-test sessions, reducing in-person counseling to 169 cases, allowing resources to be reallocated to post-test and long-term follow-up. Support strategies were tailored to life stage, including adolescent awareness, reproductive planning, and menopausal care. *Conclusion*: Comprehensive and integrated care models, including a dedicated

M. Suzuki (✉)
Center for Medical Genetics, St. Luke's International Hospital, St. Luke's International University, Chuo-ku, Tokyo, Japan
e-mail: msuzuki@luke.ac.jp

M. Arai et al. (eds.), *Practical Guide to Hereditary Breast and Ovarian Cancer IV*,
https://doi.org/10.1007/978-981-95-6580-1_7

HBOC clinic and tailored counseling, support unaffected carriers in managing hereditary cancer risk. Life-stage-based interventions and collaborative education are essential to ensure long-term surveillance and informed decision-making.

Keywords Hereditary breast and ovarian cancer · BRCA1/2 · Unaffected carriers · Genetic counseling · Risk-reducing surgery · Surveillance

1 Introduction

This paper is based on our presentation at the 4th Annual Meeting of JOHBOC and focuses on institutional practices at St. Luke's International Hospital. We report on the progress of genetic counseling and genetic testing for unaffected individuals with hereditary breast and ovarian cancer (HBOC), with particular emphasis on the dedicated HBOC clinic launched in November 2022, initially held on the fourth Saturday of each month. Since its establishment, the clinic has conducted counseling sessions with more than 350 clients, including both affected and unaffected individuals.

A distinctive feature of this clinic is the integration of same-day consultations with physicians and certified genetic counselors (CGCs). By providing separate counseling sessions in addition to medical examinations, clients are offered opportunities to explore their HBOC-related concerns in greater depth. This approach improves convenience for clients while strengthening collaboration within the multidisciplinary care team.

Drawing on this clinical experience, we highlight the psychosocial and economic burdens faced by unaffected carriers, the emotional perspectives of both affected individuals and their relatives, and the need for comprehensive support. Key issues addressed include psychological impact, financial challenges, family planning, access to clinical research, and social support needs. Through this initiative, we aim to enhance support for unaffected HBOC carriers, deepen understanding of their experiences, and contribute to improved quality of life and risk management [3, 10]. While this paper is a descriptive summary of clinical practice rather than a formal outcomes study, the experiences reported here may inform future approaches to policy and practice. It should be noted, however, that in Japan surveillance and risk-reducing surgeries for unaffected carriers remain outside the scope of national insurance, representing an important systemic limitation. While beyond the scope of this report, these observations may indicate areas where future policy development could be considered.

2 Institutional Framework and Clinical Volume

(See Table 1 for institutional surgical and genetic testing volume.) In 2023, St. Luke's International Hospital performed 877 breast cancer surgeries, including 308 mastectomies. The Center for Medical Genetics was staffed by five clinical geneticists, two Certified Nurse Specialists in Genetic Nursing (CNS, including one midwife), one Breast Cancer Nursing Certified Nurse, and two Certified Genetic Counselors (CGCs). By the end of 2023, 275 individuals had attended, with 395 cumulative visits. In 2023, a total of 16 risk-reducing mastectomies (RRMs), including two contralateral procedures, and 10 risk-reducing salpingo-oophorectomies (RRSOs) were performed at our institution. Up to 2023, a total of 153 RRMs (138 contralateral and 15 bilateral) and 198 RRSOs were performed at our institution. Based on cumulative institutional data up to 2023, occult cancer was detected in 9 of 153 risk-reducing mastectomy (RRM) cases (5.9%) and in 4 of 198 risk-reducing salpingo-oophorectomy (RRSO) cases (2.0%).

Table 1 Breakdown of genetic testing at St. Luke's International Hospital (2023)

Category	Subcategory	Number
Breast cancer, HBOC insurance	Preoperative	295
	Postoperative	58
Breast cancer, BRCACDx	Preoperative	2
	Postoperative	20
	Recurrent/metastatic	29
Breast cancer, other testing	MGPT performed	12
	BRCA-MGPT performed	4
	Self-funded BRCA	4
	BRCA-TP53 testing	3
Relatives of affected carriers	BRCA variant testing	1
Unaffected relatives	BRCA variant testing	21
Unaffected individuals	Self-funded BRCA1/2	6
	MGPT performed	11
Others	Germline findings from tumor genomic panel testing and unclassified cases	9
Total genetic tests		**475**

3 Integration with General Oncology and Screening

To facilitate early identification, intake forms were revised to capture detailed family history. Nurses confirm responses, and physicians refer patients for genetic testing or counseling. Educational sessions for staff emphasize recognition of hereditary syndromes beyond BRCA, supporting comprehensive screening and referral [3, 10].

4 Genetic Counseling Philosophy and Practice

Genetic counseling provides risk assessment, education on testing, surveillance, preventive options, and psychosocial support. Counselors guide decision-making, balancing evidence-based guidelines with patient values and preferences. Counseling also addresses family communication, enabling patients to navigate disclosure of genetic risk to relatives [6].

5 Life-Stage-Based Support

(See Table 2 for the life-stage-based support framework.) Support is tailored across the lifespan:

Weekend and evening appointments are offered to minimize disruption, enabling continuity of surveillance across life events [9].

6 Risk Awareness, Education, and Social Context

Accurate recognition of cancer risk requires integrating genetic, lifestyle, and environmental factors. Education must be collaborative. Many patients face stigma when sharing hereditary risk information with relatives. Thus, outreach extends to community education and stigma reduction. Public lectures, workshops, and professional society initiatives foster informed decision-making and family communication [7, 9]. Pancreatic surveillance with MRCP and ultrasound is also available for those with strong family histories [9].

Table 2 Life-stage-based support framework for HBOC carriers

Age group	Support and surveillance measures
Adolescence and puberty	Counseling about menstruation, HPV vaccination, breast awareness, and gene awareness
20s	Support for independence and autonomy, cancer insurance enrollment, consideration of genetic testing, cervical cancer screening, pregnancy and fertility preservation, and initiation of breast ultrasound/contrast-enhanced MRI
30s	Cervical cancer screening, pregnancy and childbirth, infertility treatment and fertility preservation, breast ultrasound/mammography/MRI, gynecologic ultrasound with CA125, and consideration of pancreatic screening
40s	Cervical and endometrial cancer screening, pregnancy/childbirth, infertility treatment and fertility preservation, breast ultrasound/mammography/MRI, consideration of RRM, gynecologic ultrasound with CA125, consideration of RRSO (with early menopause management), and consideration of abdominal ultrasound
50s	Cervical and endometrial cancer screening, management of menopausal symptoms, general cancer screening, breast ultrasound/mammography/MRI, consideration of RRM, gynecologic ultrasound with CA125, consideration of RRSO (with post-operative follow-up), and consideration of abdominal ultrasound
60s and older	Cognitive function assessment, cervical and endometrial cancer screening, management of menopausal symptoms, general cancer screening, confirmation of regular follow-up, breast ultrasound/mammography/MRI, consideration of RRM, gynecologic ultrasound with CA125, consideration of RRSO (with post-operative follow-up), and consideration of abdominal ultrasound

7 Discussion: Practical Challenges

Beyond the institutional framework and clinical outcomes, several practical challenges emerged from our HBOC clinic experience. First, the *economic burden* remains significant; some clients deferred contrast-enhanced MRI due to cost, and although clinical studies sometimes provide financial support, participation is not equally accessible to those without prior hospital attendance. Second, *convenience* is highly valued. Saturday appointments are particularly popular, and despite modest waiting times, most clients can complete breast surgery consultations, gynecologic assessments, imaging, blood sampling, and counseling within 2 hours—a system that has been positively received. Third, the clinic functions as a unique form of *psychological support*. Clients who have lost relatives to HBOC cancers often express comfort in sharing their experiences in this dedicated space, and the assurance of having at least two opportunities per year to discuss hereditary issues helps sustain long-term trust. Fourth, the need for *family-oriented support* has become increasingly apparent. Parents consider how to communicate with children about genetic risk, while caregiving responsibilities for aging relatives sometimes interfere with ongoing surveillance. Finally, issues of *fertility preservation and family planning* require dense, multidisciplinary engagement. Clients seek advice not only on preservation options but also on the timing of embryo or oocyte transfer, integration of preventive strategies such as HPV vaccination and cervical cancer screening, and the broader context of reproductive decision-making.

8 Discussion: Limitations and Novelty

While this study provides valuable insights into the management of HBOC carriers, several important limitations should be acknowledged. First, the implementation of video-based pretest counseling has not yet been formally evaluated for patient satisfaction or long-term psychological impact. Second, continuity of surveillance outside our institution remains challenging, as regional clinics may not consistently share follow-up information. Third, our analysis is based on a single institution, which may limit generalizability.

Despite these limitations, this report highlights a feature not commonly reported in Japan: the integration of an HBOC clinic within a health screening center, offering coordinated same-day consultations across multiple specialties. The life-stage–sensitive framework further emphasizes the importance of tailoring genetic counseling and risk management to patient circumstances. These innovations may serve as a reference model for similar institutions. Nevertheless, it must be acknowledged that surveillance and risk-reducing options for unaffected carriers remain uncovered by national insurance in Japan, underscoring systemic limitations. While beyond the scope of this report, these observations suggest areas where future policy development may be warranted.

9 Conclusion

St. Luke's International Hospital delivers comprehensive, stage-sensitive care for HBOC carriers. Through integrated clinics, streamlined counseling, and proactive surveillance, unaffected carriers are supported in managing cancer risk and maintaining quality of life.

Acknowledgments We thank the chairs and presenters of the 4th JOHBOC Annual Meeting for their contributions and collaboration.

Conflict of Interest The author declares no conflicts of interest related to this work.

Ethics Statement This study describes institutional practices and retrospective clinical data without identifying information. Formal ethics approval was not required according to institutional policy.

References

1. Miki Y, Swensen J, Shattuck-Eidens D, et al. A strong candidate for the breast and ovarian cancer susceptibility gene BRCA1. Science. 1994;266(5182):66–71.
2. Wooster R, Bignell G, Lancaster J, et al. Identification of the breast cancer susceptibility gene BRCA2. Nature. 1995;378(6559):789–92.
3. Daly MB, Pal T, Berry MP, et al. NCCN guidelines insights: genetic/familial high-risk assessment: breast, ovarian, and pancreatic, version 1.2022. J Natl Compr Canc Netw. 2022;20(1):38–69.
4. Rebbeck TR, Kauff ND, Domchek SM. Meta-analysis of risk reduction estimates associated with risk-reducing salpingo-oophorectomy in BRCA1 or BRCA2 mutation carriers. J Natl Cancer Inst. 2009;101(2):80–7.
5. Domchek SM, Friebel TM, Singer CF, et al. Association of risk-reducing surgery in BRCA1 or BRCA2 mutation carriers with cancer risk and mortality. JAMA. 2010;304(9):967–75.
6. Resta R, Biesecker BB, Bennett RL, et al. A new definition of genetic counseling: National Society of Genetic Counselors' Task Force report. J Genet Couns. 2006;15(2):77–83.
7. The Japanese Association of Medical Sciences. Guidelines for genetic testing and diagnosis in medical care [in Japanese]. 2011.
8. Ministry of Health, Labour and Welfare. Notification on insurance coverage for BRCA1/2 testing and risk-reducing surgery [in Japanese]. 2020.
9. Paluch-Shimon S, Cardoso F, Sessa C, et al. Prevention and screening in BRCA mutation carriers and other breast/ovarian hereditary cancer syndromes: ESMO Clinical Practice Guidelines. Ann Oncol. 2016;27(suppl 5):v103–10.
10. The Japanese Breast Cancer Society. Hereditary breast and ovarian cancer (HBOC) clinical practice guidelines, 2021 edition [in Japanese]. Tokyo: Kanehara Shuppan; 2021.

Clinical Practice for Unaffected Pathogenic Variant Carriers of *BRCA1/2*

Kanae Taruno

Abstract Unaffected carriers of pathogenic *BRCA1/2* variants comprise a high-risk population, in which timely systematic surveillance and appropriate risk-reducing interventions can markedly alter clinical trajectories. Contrast-enhanced breast magnetic resonance imaging (MRI) is the most sensitive imaging technique for the early detection of these carriers and is recommended by international guidance panels; however, real-world implementation faces policy, financial, and operational barriers that limit equitable access. This chapter proposes guidelines, presents the Showa Medical University institutional experience, details practical workflows for MRI-guided surveillance and diagnostic follow-up, summarizes outcomes and implications for treatment de-escalation, and describes risk-reducing surgical options. We also propose pragmatic steps to expand access through policy change, regional hub development, standardization of imaging practice, workforce training, and prospective studies.

Keywords Unaffected carriers · MRI · Surveillance · Risk-reduction surgery

1 Introduction

Germline pathogenic variants of *BRCA1/2* markedly increase the lifetime risk for breast and ovarian cancers and define a population in which prevention and early detection strategies are important [1]. International guidelines advocate MRI-based surveillance beginning in early adulthood and consideration of risk-reducing surgery following careful shared decision-making [2]. In Japan, diagnostic and therapeutic treatment for patients already affected by breast cancer is progressively integrated into routine practice and insurance [3]. Nonetheless, unaffected *BRCA1/2*

K. Taruno (✉)
Division of Breast Surgical Oncology, Department of Surgery, Showa Medical University School of Medicine, Tokyo, Japan
e-mail: ktaruno@med.showa-u.ac.jp

M. Arai et al. (eds.), *Practical Guide to Hereditary Breast and Ovarian Cancer IV*,
https://doi.org/10.1007/978-981-95-6580-1_8

variant carriers identified through cascade or predictive testing often face a fragmented landscape for preventive care. The availability of MRI surveillance is limited and routinely reimbursed only in certain contexts and concentrated in a small number of specialized centers. These gaps result in diagnostic delays, extensive treatments, and avoidable morbidity. This chapter draws on international recommendations and our institutional registry to discuss an operationally focused clinical guide for unaffected *BRCA1/2* carriers, which includes surveillance workflows, diagnostic follow-up for MRI-detected findings, and implementation strategies to improve access and quality of care.

2 Guidelines and Rationale for MRI-Based Surveillance

Major professional organizations recommend an enhanced surveillance strategy for *BRCA1/2* pathogenic variant carriers. The common elements include breast awareness from late adolescence, semiannual clinical breast examinations beginning in the mid-20s, and annual imaging that incorporates contrast-enhanced MRIs beginning in the mid-20s, with mammography introduced (or added) at approximately age 30 and continuing in combination with MRI through age ~75 where appropriate [2]. This guidance is supported with comparative diagnostic performance data. MRI demonstrates markedly higher sensitivity for detecting small invasive cancers, especially in younger women with dense breasts and in tumors with *BRCA*-associated biology, in which rapid growth and non-calcified features are common.

The superiority of MRI arises from its ability to visualize enhancement kinetics and morphologic features that are often occult in mammography and ultrasound images. Thus, MRI is central to surveillance designed to detect lesions at a stage that enables less extensive surgery and to avoid adjuvant systemic therapy [4]; however, the choice and timing of surveillance modalities should be individualized and account for age, reproductive plans, prior surgeries, and patient preferences.

3 Institutional Surveillance Experience of Our Institute: Methods and Cohort

Since June 2011, we have operated a prospective high-risk surveillance program. Between June 2011 and December 2022, 34 unaffected carriers were enrolled (*BRCA*1: 19; *BRCA2*: 14; male carriers: 5). Seventeen participants received comprehensive surveillance at our center, and another 13 underwent an MRI through affiliated clinical research programs or nonprofit support. The median follow-up was 36 months (range 2–96 months).

Our standard surveillance protocol combined semiannual clinical breast examinations with annual contrast-enhanced breast MRI. Mammography was included from approximately age 30 in accordance with guideline recommendations and individualized risk considerations. If a lesion was identified by MRI, we first sought a targeted second-look ultrasound. If the sonographic correlation was unavailable or inconclusive, we performed an MRI-guided vacuum-assisted core biopsy for histologic confirmation.

4 Operational Workflow and Diagnostic Pathways

Effective MRI-based surveillance requires clear operational pathways and interdepartmental coordination. Key practical components include the following:

1. Dedicated high-risk MRI capacity and reading allocation. Dedicated slots are scheduled for high-risk screening (2 weekly slots within a total of ~19 breast MRI studies/week), and a team of specialized breast MRI readers is maintained for timely interpretation and consensus review.
2. Comparative serial imaging review. Every MRI is read side-by-side along with previous studies to detect subtle morphological or kinetic changes. Incremental evolution of a small enhancing focus is an important trigger for further workup.
3. Second-look ultrasound and targeted correlation. MRI findings are routinely evaluated with targeted ultrasound to identify sonographic correlates that enable ultrasound-guided biopsy, which is faster and more comfortable for patients.
4. MRI-guided biopsy infrastructure. For MRI-only lesions, MRI-guided vacuum-assisted core biopsy is essential. Capacity constraints (approximately 1–2 MRI-guided procedures/week at our center) require judicious triage and prompt scheduling.
5. Multidisciplinary case review. MRI findings that require biopsy and confirmed malignancies are discussed at weekly multidisciplinary tumor boards, including breast surgeons, radiologists, pathologists, genetic counselors, and specialized nursing staff to ensure coordinated, patient-centered decision-making.

Based on our experience, 130 MRI-detected targets underwent biopsy (ultrasound- or MRI-guided), with an overall malignancy confirmation rate of 29%. Among *BRCA* carriers, the positive yield increased to 38%, which reflects the higher pre-test probability in this cohort and highlights the efficiency of MRI in selecting lesions for biopsy.

5 Clinical Outcomes and Implications for Treatment De-escalation

Three invasive breast cancers were detected in our cohort during surveillance. All were identified solely by MRI and were occult on contemporaneous mammography and ultrasound. Each tumor was pathologic stage pT1a or pT1b, N0. Two lesions were triple-negative (consistent with *BRCA*1 biology), and one was hormone receptor–positive. All of the cases were managed surgically with curative intent. None required adjuvant chemotherapy. These results illustrate the role of MRI in facilitating the detection of small-volume disease at a point when surgical therapy alone may suffice, thereby reducing treatment morbidity and preserving quality of life.

A representative case: A 37-year-old *BRCA*1 carrier with a strong family history was enrolled in 2015. In year seven, a routine MRI revealed a new 6-mm ring-enhancing lesion (BI-RADS 4) not visible by mammography or ultrasound. MRI-guided biopsy confirmed invasive ductal carcinoma (triple-negative). Bilateral nipple-sparing mastectomy with sentinel node biopsy (pT1aN0) was performed without adjuvant chemotherapy. At extended follow-up, she remained disease-free and is considering risk-reducing salpingo-oophorectomy (RRSO) [5].

These observations are consistent with larger cohorts showing MRI-inclusive surveillance achieves a stage shift and increases the detection of small invasive cancers in high-risk groups. The downstream effect is potentially measurable as lower systemic therapy rates and related toxicity, with favorable implications for survivorship and healthcare use if implemented broadly and equitably.

6 Risk-Reducing Surgical Options: Clinical Considerations and Implementation

Risk-reducing surgery is a core component of risk management for BRCA carriers. It encompasses bilateral risk-reducing mastectomy (BRRM) and RRSO.

Bilateral risk-reducing mastectomy (BRRM). BRRM markedly reduces the incidence of breast cancer in unaffected carriers. Although its effect on overall survival has not been definitively established, combining BRRM with adherence to other preventive measures, such as timely RRSO where indicated, contributes to comprehensive risk management [6, 7]. Candidate selection, timing, and meticulous shared decision-making are required. Considerations include age, reproductive plans, comorbidities, genetic and family history, psychosocial factors, and preferences regarding reconstruction. Reconstructive options involve implant-based (tissue expander/implant) and autologous techniques (e.g., DIEP flap), each with distinct complication profiles, recovery trajectories, and aesthetic outcomes.

Risk-reducing salpingo-oophorectomy (RRSO). RRSO is strongly recommended for BRCA1/2 carriers, typically after childbearing (commonly between ages 35 and 40). This reflects its effect in reducing ovarian/tubal cancer risk and associations with reduced all-cause and breast-cancer-specific mortality in some studies. RRSO also confers a degree of breast cancer risk reduction, which is more pronounced when performed at younger ages, although the magnitude varies based on the gene (*BRCA1* vs *BRCA2*).

Practical and financial considerations. Many risk-reducing procedures remain partially or wholly self-funded at certain centers in Japan. Preoperative evaluation out-of-pocket costs may approximate ¥150,000, whereas combined packages (bilateral mastectomy with reconstruction plus hysterectomy/adnexectomy) can reach substantial sums. For example, institutional estimates (August 2025) suggest comprehensive simultaneous procedures with a 2-week hospitalization may approach ¥1,800,000. These figures exclude potential complication-related costs. Transparent preoperative financial counseling and institution-specific cost estimates are necessary for informed consent.

Perioperative and survivorship planning. Preoperative workup should include psychosocial assessment, genetic counseling, baseline imaging, anesthetic evaluation, and addressing comorbidities. When RRSO is planned, discussions regarding menopausal symptom management, bone and cardiovascular health, and sexual function are mandatory, with long-term follow-up arrangements established.

7 Barriers to Widespread Implementation in Japan

Despite evidence supporting MRI surveillance and risk-reducing surgery, several barriers constrain implementation:

1. Insurance and reimbursement gaps. Routine MRI screening for unaffected high-risk carriers is not universally reimbursed under the current national insurance plans. Thus, many carriers must self-pay or rely on research/nonprofit support, resulting in inequitable access.
2. Facility and capacity limitations. A limited number of centers combine high-volume MRI expertise with MRI-guided biopsy capabilities. Scheduling constraints and limited procedural capacity (MRI-guided biopsies) often delay diagnosis.
3. Geographic and socioeconomic disparities. Patients living outside of major metropolitan areas can experience travel burdens and limited local access to specialist services, which compounds financial and logistical barriers.
4. Lack of standardization and training. Variability exists in MRI acquisition protocols, reporting standards, and the BI-RADS application tailored to high-risk cohorts. Targeted training programs for radiologists, technologists, and clinicians are not uniformly available.
5. Psychosocial and logistical burdens. The emotional impact of a high-risk designation, recurrent imaging appointments, and anxiety regarding invasive diagnostic procedures can reduce compliance without robust counseling and navigation support.

8 Strategic Recommendations to Improve Access and Quality

To translate evidence into population-level benefits, we propose the following multi-pronged strategy:

1. Policy advocacy for conditional coverage. Stakeholders (professional societies, academic centers, patient groups) should present consolidated evidence to national authorities (MHLW) to obtain conditional reimbursement pilots or phased coverage for MRI surveillance for unaffected BRCA carriers, accompanied by data collection on outcomes and cost-effectiveness.
2. Regional high-risk hub network. Develop designated regional hubs that provide MRI screening, MRI-guided biopsy, and multidisciplinary care, supported by tele-radiology for remote reading and second opinions to extend the reach of satellite hospitals.
3. Standardized imaging protocols and structured reporting. National consensus on MRI acquisition parameters, reporting templates, and BI-RADS use specifically tailored to variant carriers should be established and disseminated. Validation of abbreviated MRI protocols for select settings may expand capacity and preserve diagnostic yield.
4. Workforce training and credentialing. Implement targeted continuing education for MRI interpretation in *BRCA* carriers, second-look ultrasound techniques, and MRI-guided biopsy procedures. Consider formal accreditation for MRI-guided biopsy operators.
5. Integrated care pathways and patient navigation. Establish pathways that link genetic counseling, surveillance scheduling, psychosocial support, and surgical planning. Deploy patient navigators to assist with logistics, adherence, and informed decision-making.
6. Prospective research and registries. Launch prospective trials to evaluate adjuncts (e.g., ctDNA, microRNA, contrast-enhanced mammography, abbreviated MRI, chemoprevention like low-dose tamoxifen) and create national registries to monitor quality metrics (e.g., time to diagnosis, stage shift, biopsy yield, false-positive rates, adherence, treatment intensity, and costs).
7. Financial counseling and equity measures. Develop institutional policies for transparent cost disclosure, examine subsidy mechanisms for low-income patients, and integrate cost-effectiveness data into policy discussions.

9 Limitations and Implementation Considerations

Expanding MRI surveillance and risk-reducing surgery requires investment in equipment, staffing, and training. Abbreviated MRI protocols show promise for throughput and cost reduction, but require validation in *BRCA* populations, particularly younger *BRCA1* carriers with faster tumor kinetics. Any reimbursement expansion should be accompanied by quality assurance measures to prevent overuse and unnecessary biopsies. Cultural, social, and individual patient preferences should inform program design and shared decision-making processes.

10 Conclusion

MRI-inclusive surveillance is a cornerstone for early breast cancer detection in unaffected BRCA1/2 carriers, as it enables detection at stages that are amenable to less aggressive treatment. Our data demonstrate the capacity of MRI to detect small, MRI-occult tumors and to use surgical management without systemic chemotherapy in selected cases. To realize the full public health potential of these strategies, Japan must address reimbursement, capacity, standardization, and workforce challenges through coordinated policy, infrastructure, and research initiatives. In addition, providing equitable access to high-quality surveillance and well-informed risk-reducing options, including BRRM and RRSO where appropriate, will improve outcomes and reduce the burden of hereditary breast and ovarian cancer.

Competing Interests The authors have no conflicts of interest to disclose.

References

1. Kuchenbaecker KB, Hopper JL, Barnes DR, et al. Risks of breast, ovarian, and contralateral breast cancer for BRCA1 and BRCA2 mutation carriers. JAMA. 2017;317(23):2402–16.
2. Daly MB, Pal T, Maxwell KN, et al. NCCN Guidelines® insights: genetic/familial high-risk assessment: breast, ovarian, and pancreatic, version 2.2024. J Natl Compr Cancer Netw. 2023;21(10):1000–10.
3. Japan Hereditary Breast and Ovarian Cancer Comprehensive Care System Organization. Hereditary breast and ovarian cancer (HBOC) clinical practice guidelines. Kanahara Syuxtupan; 2024. xiv, 326 p.
4. Lubinski J, Kotsopoulos J, Moller P, et al. MRI surveillance and breast cancer mortality in women with BRCA1 and BRCA2 sequence variations. JAMA Oncol. 2024;10(4):493–9.
5. Mine Y, Taruno K, et al. A case of triple-negative breast cancer diagnosed by MRI-guided biopsy during surveillance of an unaffected carrier of a pathogenic *BRCA1*. Nyugan no Rinshou. 2024;39(2):161–70.
6. Li X, You R, Wang X, et al. Effectiveness of prophylactic surgeries in BRCA1 or BRCA2 mutation carriers: a meta-analysis and systematic review. Clin Cancer Res. 2016;22(15):3971–81.
7. Heemskerk-Gerritsen BAM, Jager A, Koppert LB, et al. Survival after bilateral risk-reducing mastectomy in healthy BRCA1 and BRCA2 mutation carriers. Breast Cancer Res Treat. 2019;177(3):723–33.

Issue in Unaffected Carriers from the Surveillance Outpatient Viewpoint

Yasuko Yamamoto

Abstract In 2018, the Shikoku Cancer Center established the Cancer Surveillance Clinic as a dedicated department for monitoring individuals with cancer predisposition syndromes (CPS). Notably, 30% of our patients were unaffected individuals—those without a personal history of cancer. In order to better understand the unique challenges in managing this group of patients, we have conducted a retrospective review of their clinical care. The findings revealed higher rates of clinical discontinuation and significantly lower uptake of risk-reducing salpingo-oophorectomy (RRSO) among the unaffected individuals than among those with a history of cancer. A key factor appears to be the lack of insurance coverage for CPS surveillance among unaffected individuals in Japan. However, insurance reforms alone may not be sufficient to improve engagement. The median age of the unaffected visitors was 42 years (range, 23–69 years), which is generally associated with lower cancer screening rates. This trend may reflect broader issues related to preventive health behaviors in younger populations. Many patients who discontinued care did not respond to follow-up efforts, thus suggesting a greater lack of awareness or motivation. Contributing factors may include limited public understanding of the importance of CPS surveillance, difficulty in prioritizing medical visits in the context of busy lives, and waning motivation over time. Enhancing care for this population requires not only reducing financial barriers, but also increasing public awareness of the significance of genetic risk and the role of preventive medicine in regard to CPS management.

Keywords Cancer predisposition syndrome · Cancer surveillance · Unaffected individuals · Surveillance Clinics · RRSO (risk-reducing salpingo-oophorectomy)

Y. Yamamoto (✉)
Department of Hereditary Tumors, National Hospital Organization Shikoku Cancer Center, Matsuyama, Ehime, Japan
e-mail: yamamoto.yasuko.rv@mail.hosp.go.jp

M. Arai et al. (eds.), *Practical Guide to Hereditary Breast and Ovarian Cancer IV*,
https://doi.org/10.1007/978-981-95-6580-1_9

1 Introduction

The Department of Hereditary Tumors was established at the Shikoku Cancer Center in 2000, and in August 2018, we launched the Cancer Surveillance Clinic in order to provide continuous, specialized care for individuals with cancer predisposition syndromes (CPS). The clinic was created to centralize CPS management and also facilitate long-term surveillance, particularly for unaffected individuals, for whom consistent follow-up has historically been challenging.

Several systemic issues complicate CPS surveillance in Japan. First, the financial burden was considerable. Insurance coverage for CPS-related care is highly limited, especially for unaffected individuals who are typically required to cover all out-of-pocket costs. Second, as CPS management involves multiple clinical specialties, the delineation of responsibilities among departments is often unclear, making coordinated care difficult. Third, only a few medical institutions provide dedicated CPS surveillance. Most facilities focus primarily on cancer treatment and are not structured to support the preventive care of asymptomatic individuals.

Given these barriers, the long-term follow-up of CPS surveillance is often difficult. Although individual institutions cannot resolve insurance limitations, we hypothesized that establishing a specialized clinic might help address logistical and operational challenges. Consequently, a Cancer Surveillance Clinic was established to serve as a unified access point for CPS-related surveillance.

Our clinic accepts a broad range of patients, including those with CPS confirmed via genetic testing, individuals suspected of having CPS despite negative test results, those with variants of uncertain significance (VUS), and patients who have not undergone genetic testing but have strong clinical indicators of hereditary cancer risk. Surveillance protocols were based on both domestic and international guidelines [1–4]. Although risk-reducing salpingo-oophorectomy (RRSO) for hereditary breast and ovarian cancer (HBOC) is generally limited to designated hospitals under the Japanese insurance system, we developed an infrastructure to provide RRSO on a self-pay basis at our institution.

More than 5 years after the launch of the clinic, we have conducted a retrospective review of clinical practices, focusing particularly on the unique challenges associated with the management of unaffected individuals with CPS.

2 Method

We retrospectively analyzed 182 individuals who visited the Cancer Surveillance Clinic between September 2018 and March 2024. Clinical data were extracted from medical records and included the following variables: personal cancer history, implementation and results of genetic testing, incidence of new cancers after initiating clinic visits, continuation or discontinuation of surveillance, and performance of risk-reducing salpingo-oophorectomies (RRSO).

For cases in which clinic attendance was discontinued, the reasons for discontinuation were reviewed and categorized based on documentation in the medical records. We classified the reasons into two categories: (1) acceptable reasons (e.g., death and relocation) and (2) concerning reasons (e.g., financial burden, personal decisions, or failure to attend scheduled appointments without communication).

3 Results

3.1 Patient Characteristics

Between September 2018 and March 2024, 182 individuals visited the Cancer Surveillance Clinic, including 138 affected (those with a personal history of cancer) and 44 unaffected individuals. The median age at the initial visit was 51.5 years (range, 27–76 years) for affected individuals and 44 years (range, 23–68 years) for unaffected individuals (Table 1). Some patients underwent genetic testing prior to 2018.

Among the 44 unaffected individuals, 8 did not undergo genetic testing. Of the 36 tested cases, more than half carried pathogenic variants of BRCA1 or BRCA2. Five individuals had no pathogenic variants, and one had a variant of uncertain significance (VUS). In the affected group, only one individual did not undergo genetic testing. The distribution of pathogenic variants was similar to that in the unaffected group, with BRCA1/2 mutations accounting for the majority (Fig. 1).

Since partial insurance coverage for HBOC was introduced in 2020, 32 unaffected individuals have been newly diagnosed with CPS at our institution. Of these, 22 underwent cancer surveillance. Among the 10 individuals who did not, eight were either under the recommended age for surveillance or declined participation. As a result, 22 of the 24 eligible cases (91.7%) commenced surveillance despite being ineligible for insurance coverage.

Table 1 Clinical characteristics of patients at the Cancer Surveillance Clinic

	Unaffected individuals (n = 44)	Affected individuals (n = 138)
Sex		
Female	41	137
Male	3	1
Age at genetic testing, median [range]	45.0[a] (23–67)	50.0[b] (27–76)
Age at first visit to the Cancer Surveillance Clinic, median [range]	44.0 (23–68)	51.5 (27–76)

[a]Nine cases without genetic testing were excluded from this analysis
[b]The two cases that had not undergone genetic testing were excluded

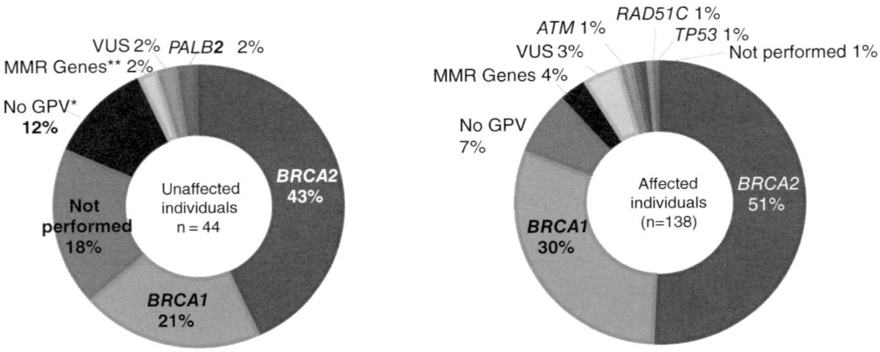

Fig. 1 Distribution of genes with pathogenic variants detected in patients at the Cancer Surveillance Clinic. *No GPV: No germline pathogenic variants detected. **MMR genes: *MLH1*, *MSH2*, *PMS2*, and *MSH6*

Table 2 Patients diagnosed with new cancers during surveillance

	Genes with pathological variants	Affected cancer type	Cancer diagnosed after surveillance began	Age at diagnosis	Triggering test
Unaffected individuals	*BRCA2*	–	Breast cancer	41	MRI
	BRCA2	–	Breast cancer	53	MRI
	BRCA2	–	Breast cancer	42	MRI
Affected individuals	*TP53*	Osteosarcoma	Breast cancer	28	MRI
	BRCA2	Breast cancer	Bladder cancer Fallopian tube cancer Vaginal cancer	72	–
	BRCA2	Breast cancer	Gastric cancer	60	EGD[a]
	PALB2 (VUS)	Breast cancer	Fallopian tube cancer	79	Serum CA125

[a]Esophagogastroduodenoscopy

3.2 *Incidence of New Cancer During Surveillance*

During the observation period, seven individuals developed new cancer: four in the affected group and three in the unaffected group (Table 2).

3.3 *Discontinuation of Clinic Visits*

Of these 182 individuals, 31 discontinued clinic attendance. The discontinuation rate was 13% (17/138) in the affected group and 28% (14/44) in the unaffected group, indicating a notably higher dropout rate among the unaffected individuals.

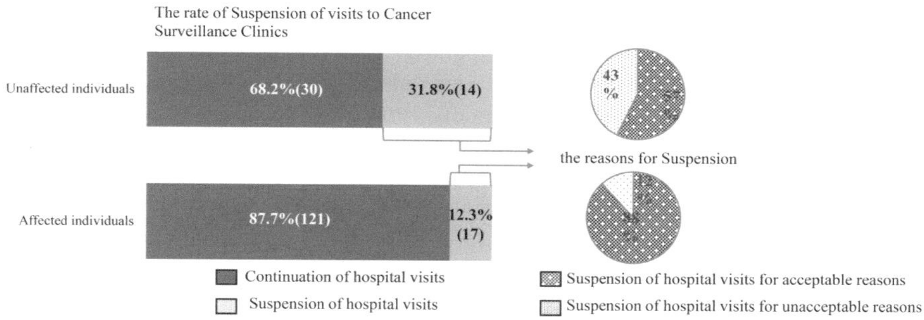

Fig. 2 Rates and reasons for clinic visit discontinuation among affected and unaffected individuals

Reasons for discontinuation were categorized as either acceptable (e.g., death or relocation) or concerning (e.g., personal choice, financial difficulty, or missed appointments). The reasons accounted for 11.8% (2/17) of the affected individuals and 42.9% (6/14) of the unaffected individuals. Among the eight cases classified according to the following reasons, six failed to attend scheduled appointments and did not return despite follow-up contact (Fig. 2).

3.4 Implementation of Risk-Reducing Salpingo-Oophorectomy (RRSO)

Among the individuals with elevated genetic risk for ovarian cancer (including genes beyond BRCA1/2), the RRSO implementation rate was 39.8% (74/186) in the affected group and 8.5% (4/47) in the unaffected group.

4 Discussion

Several challenges hinder the effective delivery of care for individuals with cancer predisposition syndrome (CPS) in Japan. These include insufficient infrastructure for genetic counseling and cancer surveillance, limited insurance coverage, and a general lack of public awareness of hereditary cancer syndromes. Among these, the lack of insurance coverage for unaffected individuals is particularly pressing.

Although partial insurance coverage for hereditary breast and ovarian cancers (HBOC) was introduced in 2020, it remains limited to affected individuals. Unaffected individuals continue to bear the full cost of surveillance, raising long-standing concerns about adherence to and continuity of care. Given that CPS care is not yet widely adopted in Japan, the fact that unaffected individuals proactively visit specialized clinics may indicate a high awareness and motivation for cancer prevention in this population.

Previous studies on the general population have shown that individuals with close relatives affected by cancer are more likely to undergo cancer screening because of their heightened awareness and perceived personal risk [5]. Naghi et al. in their study reported that carriers of pathogenic variants in BRCA1/2 or other high-risk genes were approximately 10 times more likely to undergo MRI surveillance than low-risk individuals, thus demonstrating the strong influence of genetic risk perception on preventive behavior.

Consistent with these findings, approximately 90% of the unaffected individuals diagnosed with CPS at our institution initiated surveillance despite the absence of insurance coverage. However, the discontinuation rate remained high at 28%, which was more than double that of affected individuals (13%). This discrepancy highlights the unique difficulty in sustaining long-term engagement among asymptomatic individuals, even when the initial motivation is strong.

The low rate of risk-reducing salpingo-oophorectomy (RRSO) in unaffected individuals was particularly striking. Although the preventive benefits of RRSO in HBOC are well established, Kahn et al. reported an approximately 80% reduction in ovarian cancer risk and a potential 15% decrease in mortality through widespread implementation [6]; however, the uptake among our unaffected patients remained at only 8.5%. This finding reflects the significant gap in the translation of genetic risk information into concrete preventive measures.

The most substantial barrier for unaffected individuals is arguably the structural barrier. Japan's universal health insurance system generally prohibits mixed billing, which restricts the ability of insured medical institutions to provide additional self-paying services. Consequently, many facilities are unable to offer surveillance services to unaffected individuals, thereby limiting geographical and institutional access. Furthermore, a shortage of trained genetic specialists exacerbates this limitation, with few institutions providing comprehensive CPS care.

Beyond institutional constraints, broader social factors are likely to contribute to poor follow-up among unaffected individuals. Although this study did not include qualitative interviews, our findings suggest that many patients, particularly younger individuals, face competing demands from work, family, and other responsibilities. Without visible symptoms or a prior cancer diagnosis, it may be difficult for these patients to prioritize regular surveillance. Social norms and limited public awareness of hereditary cancers may further reduce the perceived urgency of such care.

Improving care for unaffected individuals with CPS requires a two-pronged approach: system-level reform and societal engagement. Expanding insurance coverage is essential, but insufficient on its own. Broad public education efforts are needed to normalize preventive medicine based on genetic risk and to ensure that individuals understand both their personal risks and the long-term benefits of surveillance.

From a medical standpoint, additional challenges include the development of standardized evidence-based surveillance protocols. Most current practices are designed around HBOC, for which risk-reducing interventions are well supported by the data. However, the increased use of multigene panel testing (MGPT) has identified individuals with variants in less well-characterized genes for whom evidence-based guidelines are lacking. Future research must therefore address these gaps to support informed decision-making.

Finally, CPS care must be dynamic and responsive to the changing life stages. A seamless, multidisciplinary follow-up system is especially important for patients in the adolescent and young adult (AYA) generation to address needs such as pregnancy planning, surgical menopause following RRSO, and family inheritance. We can improve long-term outcomes for unaffected individuals at high genetic risk only through coordinated efforts across the medical, institutional, and societal domains.

References

1. National Comprehensive Cancer Network: NCCN Clinical Practice Guidelines in Oncology. Genetic/familial high-risk assessment: breast, ovarian, pancreatic, and prostate. Version 3.2025. https://www.nccn.org/professionals/physician_gls/pdf/genetics_bopp.pdf.
2. National Comprehensive Cancer Network: NCCN Clinical Practice Guidelines in Oncology. Genetic/familial high-risk assessment: colorectal, endometrial, and gastric. Version 4.2024. https://www.nccn.org/professionals/physician_gls/pdf/genetics_ceg.pdf.
3. Japan Organization of Hereditary Breast and Ovarian Cancer. Guidelines for diagnosis and treatment of hereditary breast and ovarian cancer. 2024. https://johboc.jp/guidebook_2024/.
4. JSCCR guidelines 2024 for the clinical practice of hereditary colorectal cancer. Japanese Society for Cancer of the Colon and Rectum.
5. Akiyama M, Ishida N, Takahashi H, Takahashi M, Otsuki A, Sato Y, Saito J, Yaguchi-Saito A, Fujimori M, Kaji Y, Shimazu T. Screening practices of cancer survivors and individuals whose family or friends had a cancer diagnoses-a nationally representative cross-sectional survey in Japan (INFORM Study 2020). J Cancer Surviv. 2023;17(3):663–76. https://doi.org/10.1007/s11764-023-01367-4.
6. Naghi LA, Culver JO, Ricker C, Sturgeon D, Kingham K, Hodan R, et al. Breast cancer MRI screening of patients after multiplex gene panel testing. JAMA Netw Open. 2025;8(1):e2454447. https://doi.org/10.1001/jamanetworkopen.2024.54447.

Present Status of Clinical Practice for HBOC Carriers Without Ovarian Cancer

Hidetaka Nomura

Abstract *Background*: Hereditary breast and ovarian cancer (HBOC) caused by pathogenic variants in *BRCA1/2* genes confers a markedly elevated lifetime risk of ovarian and breast cancers. While risk-reducing salpingo-oophorectomy (RRSO) remains the only proven preventive strategy for tubo-ovarian cancer, public health insurance coverage in Japan currently extends only to breast cancer survivors, leaving unaffected carriers without financial support. *Methods*: We reviewed the impact of the introduction of public insurance coverage for RRSO at the Cancer Institute Hospital and described our institutional surveillance protocol for *BRCA1/2* pathogenic variant carriers who defer RRSO. The protocol incorporates serum CA125 measurement and transvaginal ultrasonography every 3 months, supplemented by endometrial cytology every 6 months. *Results*: Following the implementation of insurance coverage in April 2020, the annual number of RRSO procedures increased 3.9-fold, with shorter intervals between HBOC diagnosis and surgery. Surveillance identified five cases of ovarian or fallopian tube cancer, two of which were triggered by positive endometrial cytology. Importantly, complete macroscopic resection (R0) was achieved in all cases, despite diagnoses at FIGO stage III. *Conclusion*: Our experience highlights the clinical utility of integrating endometrial cytology into HBOC surveillance and suggests that surveillance may facilitate R0 resection even in advanced-stage cases. Nonetheless, the current restriction of RRSO insurance coverage to breast cancer survivors imposes significant inequity. Expanding coverage to unaffected carriers is essential for equitable care, timely preventive intervention, and improved oncologic outcomes in Japan.

Keywords Hereditary breast and ovarian cancer (HBOC) · *BRCA1/2* · Risk-reducing salpingo-oophorectomy (RRSO) · Public health insurance · Ovarian cancer surveillance · Endometrial cytology

H. Nomura (✉)
Department of Gynecology, Cancer Institute Hospital of Japanese Foundation for Cancer Research, Tokyo, Japan
e-mail: hidetaka.nomura@jfcr.or.jp

M. Arai et al. (eds.), *Practical Guide to Hereditary Breast and Ovarian Cancer IV*,
https://doi.org/10.1007/978-981-95-6580-1_10

1 Background and Outline of Public Insurance Coverage

Genetic testing for *BRCA1/2* and risk-reducing salpingo-oophorectomy (RRSO) were incorporated into the Japanese public health insurance system in April 2020. Before this, these interventions would be offered as self-financed medical services. This would impose a substantial financial burden on patients, and some patients would be compelled to forgo testing or surgery for economic reasons.

Since April 2020, genetic testing, though limited to women with a prior diagnosis of breast or ovarian cancer, is reimbursed by public health insurance, with the reimbursement fee being set at 20,200 points. As an institutional requirement, facilities were required to be registered to claim the genetic counseling surcharge. However, the presence of a dedicated department of clinical genetics was not mandatory. Institutions that had not submitted such registration could also claim reimbursement, provided they had collaborated with accredited facilities and had ensured the provision of appropriate genetic counseling.

With regard to risk-reducing surgery, procedures performed on patients with hereditary breast and ovarian cancer at institutions that had been formally registered with the Regional Bureau of Health and Welfare were reimbursable. It was mandatory to convene a multidisciplinary conference including specialists in clinical genetics as well as breast surgeons or gynecologic oncologists, to discuss treatment strategies based on the results of genetic counseling, prior to the surgery. Furthermore, as prerequisites for reimbursement under the public insurance scheme, it was necessary to thoroughly inform the patients about the purpose of the procedure, as well as the associated benefits and risks.

2 Institutional Experience: Changes Before and After Insurance Coverage at the Cancer Institute Hospital

A retrospective analysis of the clinical impact of the introduction of public insurance coverage for RRSO, including *BRCA1/2* pathogenic variant carriers who underwent RRSO between January 2017 and December 2022, was conducted at our institution [1]. Patients were stratified into two cohorts: the pre-coverage period (January 2017–March 2020: Period A) and the post-coverage period (April 2020–December 2022: Period B).

Overall, 134 women underwent RRSO at our institution during the study period. The baseline characteristics of Periods A and B are summarized in Table 1. In Period A, 45 women underwent RRSO in 36 months, whereas 89 women underwent RRSO in 24 months in Period B. The median age, *BRCA* status, personal breast cancer history, and family history of ovarian cancer within the third degree were not statistically different. In Period B, there were significantly more parous women. Four women who had been waiting for the introduction of public insurance underwent RRSO at the early stage of Period B. After the introduction of public insurance

Table 1 Clinical characteristics of BRCA pathogenic variant carriers undergoing RRSO (Period A vs Period B)

	Total	Period A		Period B		
		BRCA1	*BRCA2*	*BRCA1*	*BRCA2*	*p*-value
BRCA pathogenic variant carriers	134	45		89		<0.001
		27 (60%)	18 (40%)	47 (52.8%)	42 (47.2%)	0.54
Median age at RRSO (range)	48.5 (38–74)	50 (38–74)		48 (32–73)		0.12
Personal breast cancer history	122	39 (86.7%)		83 (93.3%)		0.35
Familial history of ovarian cancer third-degree relatives	53	16 (35.6%)		33 (37.1%)		1
Parous	99	28 (62.2%)		71 (79.8%)		0.048
Paid by insurance						
No	51	45 (100%)		6 (6.7%)		<0.01
Yes	83	0		83 (93.3%)		
Number per month		1.25		3.71		<0.01

Table 2 Genetic testing performed in each group

	Period A		Period B	
	Number	Positive	Number	Positive
BRACAnalysis	245	25 (10.2%)	1720	188 (10.9%)
Breast cancer	180	13 (7.8%)	1288	110 (8.5%)
Ovarian cancer	65	11 (16.9%)	249	64 (25.7%)
Pancreatic cancer	0	0	112	8 (7.1%)
Prostate cancer	0	0	71	6 (8.5%)
Other genetic tests for HBOC	132	23 (17.4%)	2	1 (50%)
Total	377	48 (12.7%)	1722	189 (11.0%)
Number per month	10.5	1.33	71.8	7.88

coverage, a 3.0-fold increase was observed in the annual number of RRSO procedures. This change in policy enabled patients to undergo RRSO concomitantly with breast cancer surgery performed under the coverage of the public insurance system. In addition, a shorter interval between hereditary breast and ovarian cancer diagnosis and RRSO facilitated preventive intervention at more appropriate time points [2].

Genetic testing was performed in 377 women in Period A and 1722 women in Period B in our hospital (Table 2). The number of women diagnosed with *BRCA* pathogenic variants increased 3.9-fold (189/48) in Period B compared with Period A. Furthermore, there was a 5.9-fold (7.88/1.33) increase in the number of women with positive genetic testing per month in Period B.

These findings indicate that insurance coverage alleviated financial barriers and stabilized clinical practice through systematization, thereby expanding access. The conclusion of the analysis was that this policy reform would promote equitable access to HBOC care across Japan and contribute to improved oncologic outcomes.

3 Background of the Surveillance Protocol

The most reliable strategy for primary prevention of tubo-ovarian cancer in *BRCA1/2* pathogenic variant carriers is the RRSO. However, surveillance is often proposed as an interim strategy for patients who have not yet reached the recommended age for RRSO or for those who choose to defer the timing of surgery.

While early detection is crucial for improving the prognosis of cancer patients, in HBOC, ovarian cancers are frequently diagnosed at advanced stages. The limitations in both sensitivity and specificity of traditional surveillance modalities such as serum CA125 measurement and transvaginal ultrasonography (TVUS) make early detection of precursor lesions difficult. In recent years, pathological studies have confirmed the origin of most high-grade serous carcinomas (HGSCs) from epithelial lesions of the fimbrial end of the fallopian tube, specifically serous tubal intraepithelial carcinoma (STIC). This finding highlights the clinical importance of the detection of early tubal lesions.

Based on these insights, a surveillance protocol incorporating endometrial cytology was designed by our institution for enhancing sensitivity compared with conventional methods and for detecting early precancerous or microscopic tubal lesions.

4 Outline of Our Institutional Protocol

The surveillance protocol at our institution, for *BRCA1/2* pathogenic variant carriers, consists of serum CA125 measurement every 3 months, transvaginal ultrasonography every 3 months, and endometrial cytology every 6 months [3].

Endometrial cytology can occasionally detect neoplastic cells of tubal origin that exfoliate into the endometrial cavity, though it has traditionally been employed as a screening tool for endometrial carcinoma. This is particularly relevant since HBOC-related ovarian cancers are now known to frequently arise from the fimbrial end of the fallopian tube. Indeed, we have diagnosed STIC by endometrial cytology in our clinical experience [4] and have therefore integrated endometrial cytology into our ovarian cancer surveillance strategy for women with HBOC.

5 Objectives of Surveillance

In women with HBOC, ovarian cancer is often diagnosed at an advanced stage, with the majority of cases presenting as FIGO stage III or higher at diagnosis. The 5-year survival rate for stage III ovarian cancer, underscoring the poor prognosis, has been reported to be only 30%–40%. However, a significant improvement in prognosis has been observed when complete macroscopic resection (R0) is achieved during primary surgery [5, 6]. Achieving R0 cytoreduction enhances the effectiveness of adjuvant chemotherapy by reducing the tumor burden, thereby prolonging progression-free survival, and potentially improving overall survival [7].

Early detection, particularly in stage III disease, remains difficult; however, identifying tumors when the extent of dissemination is still limited is clinically meaningful. Previous studies have demonstrated that surveillance of *BRCA* pathogenic variant carriers rarely enables diagnosis at an early stage [8]. Therefore, the realistic objective of surveillance in this high-risk population is diagnosis at a stage when complete resection remains feasible, rather than prevention of advanced stage presentation.

6 Surveillance Outcomes at the Cancer Institute Hospital

A retrospective analysis of the outcomes of surveillance among *BRCA1/2* pathogenic variant carriers at our institution, with a particular focus on cases of ovarian and fallopian tube cancer, was conducted, with the surveillance protocol consisting of CA125 measurement every 3 months, transvaginal ultrasonography every 3 months, and endometrial cytology every 6 months, as mentioned earlier.

A total of five cases of ovarian or fallopian tube cancer were diagnosed through surveillance during the study period (Table 3). In two cases, positive endometrial cytology was the key diagnostic trigger. Importantly, complete macroscopic resection (R0) was achieved in every patient, despite all cases being diagnosed at FIGO stage III.

Among the five cases, histopathological examination revealed four cases of HGSC and one case of carcinosarcoma. Either the fimbrial end of the fallopian tube or the ovaries were identified as the primary sites. All patients underwent postoperative chemotherapy, and short-term outcomes indicated disease-free survival in all cases.

This study indicates that though surveillance does not eliminate the risk of advanced stage presentation, it might facilitate diagnosis at a stage with lower tumor

Table 3 Clinical characteristics of tubo-ovarian cancer cases detected through surveillance

	Case 1	Case 2	Case 3	Case 4	Case 5
Age at ovarian cancer diagnosis, years	62	64	51	47	49
Causative gene	*BRCA1*	*BRCA1*	*BRCA1*	*BRCA1*	*BRCA1*
CA125 (U/mL)	96	168	Not measured	6	3
Transvaginal ultrasonography	Normal	Swollen right ovary	Ascites	Swollen left ovary	Normal
Endometrial cytology	Positive	Negative	Positive	Negative	Negative
Stage	Stage IIIB	Stage IIIB	Stage IIIC	Stage IIIB	Stage IIIC

burden, thereby increasing the likelihood of achieving R0 resection and potentially improving patient prognosis.

7 Background of Insurance Coverage and Current Framework

Multiple studies have previously demonstrated that RRSO significantly reduces the risk of ovarian and fallopian tube cancer among *BRCA1/2* pathogenic variant carriers. RRSO was incorporated into the public health insurance system in Japan in April 2020; however, eligibility was restricted to women with a prior history of breast cancer, rendering unaffected carriers ineligible for reimbursement. Unaffected women wishing to undergo RRSO are required to bear the entire cost out-of-pocket. At our institution, the expense for bilateral salpingo-oophorectomy is around 750,000 JPY, while bilateral salpingo-oophorectomy combined with hysterectomy costs around 1,050,000 JPY, which includes preoperative evaluations, hospitalization, and surgery.

In addition, the out-of-pocket expenses for surveillance are not negligible when public insurance coverage is not applied. At our institution, the surveillance program for *BRCA1/2* pathogenic variant carriers consists of serum CA125 measurement every 3 months (4510 JPY at full charge, 1353 JPY with 30% copayment), transvaginal ultrasonography every 3 months (5300 JPY/1590 JPY), and endometrial cytology every 6 months (6500 JPY/1950 JPY). In addition, annual cervical cytology (1900 JPY/570 JPY) and follow-up consultation fees every 3 months (730 JPY/219 JPY) are required. When calculated in total, the annual expense amounts to approximately 140,000 JPY on a self-financed basis, including all examinations and follow-up visits.

8 Regional Disparities During the Era of Self-Financed Care

Prior to being covered by public insurance, RRSO was largely limited to specialized centers in urban areas. Twenty-three (13.8%) and 14 (8.4%) facilities were located in Tokyo and Osaka, respectively. Furthermore, 74 (44.3%) facilities were in three megalopolises in Tokyo (Tokyo, Kanagawa, Chiba, and Saitama), Osaka (Osaka, Kyoto, and Hyogo), and Nagoya (Aichi) [9]. In order to access surgical services, patients living in rural regions were often required to travel long distances, mostly requiring overnight stays. Furthermore, the inadequacy of the local availability of genetic counseling and postoperative follow-up highlights the lack of equity in HBOC care prior to systematization.

9 Limitations of the Current System: Exclusion of Unaffected Carriers

The number of RRSO procedures in breast cancer survivors has markedly increased following the introduction of insurance coverage. However, the persistent economic and geographic barriers result in limited uptake among unaffected carriers. While the essence of preventive medicine lies in pre-symptomatic intervention, despite their clearly elevated risk identified through family history or genetic testing, the unaffected women are denied access by the current framework. Consequently, these individuals face substantial financial burdens, and many are forced to abandon the option of surgery at the optimal timing.

10 Long-Term Consequences of Self-Financed Procedures

RRSO performed as a self-financed procedure is associated with a serious problem. Public insurance excludes coverage for subsequent medical care for complications or sequelae as per the current regulations. This is similar to cases observed in Japan, where individuals who underwent self-financed liver transplantation abroad and later developed hepatitis were denied coverage for subsequent treatment under the national insurance scheme. In other words, when a patient elects to undergo a self-financed intervention, any subsequent healthcare issues related to that procedure will also be permanently excluded from insurance reimbursement, resulting in a sustained financial burden. This systemic barrier can lead to patient–provider conflicts in the event of postoperative complications.

11 Future Perspectives

Expanding insurance coverage of RRSO to unaffected *BRCA1/2* pathogenic variant carriers is essential to reduce the incidence of ovarian cancer and improve survival outcomes, as well as to ensure equity within the healthcare system. The current framework represents only an initial step. Moving forward, comprehensive coverage should include risk-reducing surgery as well as genetic testing for high-risk women. Furthermore, establishing nationwide systems that guarantee access to genetic counseling and surgical expertise throughout Japan, including the rural regions, will be critical for improving outcomes in HBOC management in Japan.

References

1. Nomura H, Abe A, Fusegi A, et al. Impact of the coverage of risk-reducing salpingo-oophorectomy by the national insurance system for women with *BRCA* pathogenic variants in Japan. Sci Rep. 2023;13(1):1018. https://doi.org/10.1038/s41598-023-28304-w.
2. Abe A, Nomura H, Fusegi A, et al. Risk-reducing decisions regarding germline *BRCA* pathogenic variant: focusing on the timing of genetic testing and RRSO. J Med Genet. 2024;61(4):392–8. https://doi.org/10.1136/jmg-2023-109549.
3. Fusegi A, Nomura H, Ueki A, et al. Ovarian surveillance including endometrial cytology for patients with hereditary breast and ovarian cancer before risk-reducing salpingo-oophorectomy: a retrospective analysis. J Obstet Gynaecol Res. 2024;50(6):1002–9. https://doi.org/10.1111/jog.15935.
4. Nomura H, Abe A, Yamamoto A, et al. A case of recurrent fallopian tube carcinoma in situ with para-aortic lymph node metastasis. Int Cancer Conf J. 2013;2:161–4. https://doi.org/10.1007/s13691-013-0082-1.
5. Wallace S, Kumar A, McGree M, et al. Efforts at maximal cytoreduction improve survival in ovarian cancer patients, even when complete gross resection is not feasible. Gynecol Oncol. 2017;45:21–6. https://doi.org/10.1016/j.ygyno.2017.01.029.
6. Du Bois A, Reuss A, Pujade-Lauraine E, et al. Role of surgical outcome as prognostic factor in advanced epithelial ovarian cancer: a combined exploratory analysis of 3 prospectively randomized phase 3 multicenter trials: by the Arbeitsgemeinschaft Gynaekologische Onkologie Studiengruppe Ovarialkarzinom (AGO-OVAR) and the Groupe d'Investigateurs Nationaux Pour les Etudes des Cancers de l'Ovaire (GINECO). Cancer. 2009;115(6):1234–44. https://doi.org/10.1002/cncr.24149.
7. Bristow RE, Tomacruz RS, Armstrong DK, et al. Survival effect of maximal cytoreductive surgery for advanced ovarian carcinoma during the platinum era: a meta-analysis. J Clin Oncol. 2002;20:1248–59. https://doi.org/10.1200/JCO.2002.20.5.1248.
8. Rosenthal AN. Ovarian cancer screening in the high-risk population—the UK Familial Ovarian Cancer Screening Study (UKFOCSS). Int J Gynecol Cancer. 2012;22:S27–8. https://doi.org/10.1097/IGC.0b013e318251cc3f.
9. Hirayama T, Inayama Y, Odajima S, et al. A report on the 73th Annual Congress of the Japan Society of Obstetrics and Gynecology International Workshop for Junior Fellows: risk-reducing surgery for hereditary breast and ovarian cancer. J Obstet Gynaecol Res. 2021;47(11):3761–6. https://doi.org/10.1111/jog.14952.

Equalization and Regional Cooperation of Clinical Practice for Hereditary Tumor

Proliferation and Regional Cooperation in HBOC Clinical Practice

Tomoyuki Aruga

Abstract Breast cancer is the most frequently diagnosed malignancy among Japanese women, yet gaps in early detection persist, and a substantial proportion of patients present with stage II or higher disease. Germline susceptibility—dominated by BRCA1/2—accounts for a meaningful fraction of cases, with higher prevalence in younger age, bilateral disease, and triple-negative phenotypes, and several variants enriched within the Japanese population. Over the past decade, Japan's public insurance coverage has progressively incorporated BRCA1/2 testing—first as a companion diagnostic and later for hereditary breast and ovarian cancer (HBOC) diagnosis—while professional societies have established coordinated frameworks for education, guidelines, databases, and workforce training. Building on this foundation, we propose embedding HBOC-appropriate genetic testing within community breast clinics at the time of diagnosis to inform surgical planning and perioperative PARP inhibitor eligibility, shorten turnaround-related delays, and enable secondary screening of previously treated patients. Practical implementation requires compliance notifications, structured referral pathways with core hospitals and genetics units, and accredited staff training; a regional network model in Tokyo demonstrates feasibility. Key challenges include reimbursement lags, administrative burden, immediate counseling needs after a new cancer diagnosis, and difficulty staffing genetics-trained personnel in small practices. Strengthening clinic–tertiary center collaboration and providing institutional support are essential to deliver timely, accurate, and equitable HBOC services nationwide.

Keywords Hereditary breast and ovarian cancer (HBOC) · BRCA1/2 · Genetic testing · Clinic-based care · Regional collaboration

---

T. Aruga (✉)
Department of Surgical Specialties, Institute of Science Tokyo, Tokyo, Japan

Department of Breast Surgery/Clinical Genetics, Tokyo Metropolitan Cancer and Infectious Disease Center, Komagome Hospital, Tokyo, Japan

M. Arai et al. (eds.), *Practical Guide to Hereditary Breast and Ovarian Cancer IV*, https://doi.org/10.1007/978-981-95-6580-1_11

1 Current Status of Breast Cancer in Japan

Breast cancer is now the most frequently diagnosed malignancy among Japanese women. In 2021, approximately 94,000 women were newly diagnosed, and about 15,000 died of the disease; breast cancer accounted for 22.6% of all malignancies in women [1]. The Japanese Breast Cancer Society registry recorded 98,540 cases that year from more than 1300 institutions, with a median diagnostic age in the 50 s and the highest proportions among women aged 45–49 (13.5%) and 70–74 (13.3%) [2]. Early-stage disease (stage 0–I) comprised 57.6% of cases, yet roughly 40% were diagnosed at stage II or beyond, indicating persistent gaps in early detection. A family history of breast cancer was reported in 18.5% of patients. Diagnoses before age 40 made up 4.4%, and bilateral disease—metachronous or synchronous—accounted for 11.3%; both groups warrant thorough hereditary breast and ovarian cancer (HBOC) assessment in clinical evaluation.

2 *BRCA1/2* Variants in the Japanese Population

Germline pathogenic variants in *BRCA1/2* are enriched in early-onset breast cancer, bilateral disease, and cases with ovarian cancer. In a large Japanese case–control study evaluating 11 susceptibility genes in 7051 unselected patients, pathogenic variants were detected in 5.7%; approximately two-thirds were *BRCA1/2*, underscoring their central role in genetic susceptibility (Table 1) [3]. *BRCA1/2*

Table 1 Result of gene-based association test using pathogenic variants

Gene	No. of pathogenic variants	Case (n = 7051) No. of carriers (%)	Control (n = 11,241) No. of carriers (%)	P-value[a]	OR	(95% CI)
BRCA2	85	191 (2.71)	19 (0.17)	9.87×10^{-58}	16.4	(10.2–28.0)
BRCA1	55	102 (1.45)	5 (0.04)	3.71×10^{-36}	33.0	(13.7–103.8)
PALB2	21	28 (0.40)	5 (0.04)	5.79×10^{-8}	9.0	(3.4–29.7)
TP53	13	16 (0.23)	3 (0.03)	5.93×10^{-5}	8.5	(2.4–45.6)
PTEN	12	11 (0.16)	1 (0.01)	2.16×10^{-4}	17.6	(2.6–753.3)
CHEK2	17	26 (0.37)	13 (0.12)	4.31×10^{-4}	3.2	(1.6–6.8)
NF1	8	8 (0.11)	0 (0.00)	4.86×10^{-4}	Inf	(2.7–Inf)
ATM	27	22 (0.31)	17 (0.15)	0.031	2.1	(1.0–4.1)
CDH1	2	2 (0.03)	0 (0.00)	0.149	Inf	(0.3–Inf)
NBN	3	1 (0.01)	3 (0.03)	1.000	0.5	(0.0–6.6)
STK11	1	0 (0.00)	1 (0.01)	1.000	0.0	(0.0–62.1)
Sum	**244**	**404[b] (5.73)**	**67 (0.60)**	$\mathbf{2.87 \times 10^{-102}}$	**10.1**	**(7.8–13.4)**

Momozawa et al. [3]
[a]Fisher's exact test
[b]Sum of carriers from the 11 genes was 407. However, three patients had two pathogenic variants in different genes. Thus, the number of carriers became 404

prevalence varied markedly by age (e.g., 15.0% <40 years vs. 3.2% ≥80 years), and *BRCA1* variants were strongly associated with triple-negative disease, younger age, and bilateral cancer (Fig. 1). Another analysis of 1406 counseled patients reported a 9.4% rate of pathogenic *BRCA1/2* variants, with higher frequencies among younger individuals and those with bilateral disease [4]. Several variants appear to be enriched or unique in the Japanese population, supporting the need for population-tailored risk assessment and personalized care.

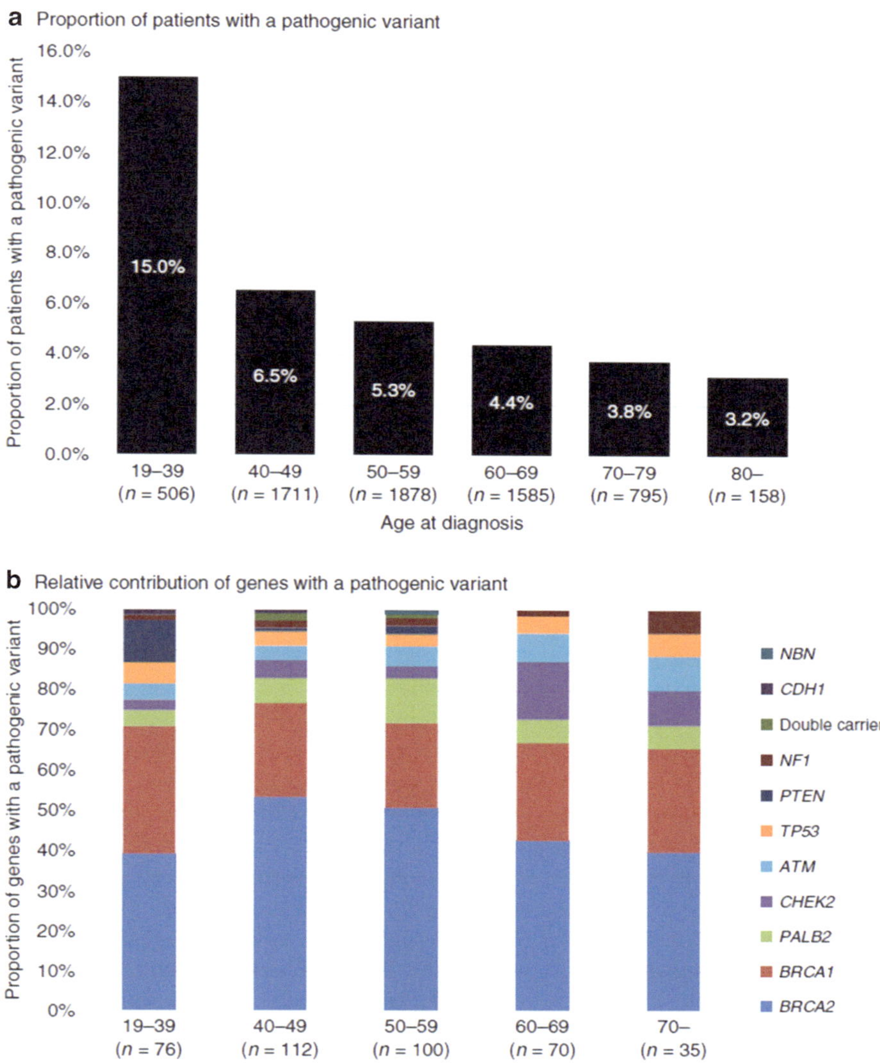

Nat Commun. 2018 Oct 4;9(1):4083.

Fig. 1 (**a**) Proportion of patients with pathogenic variants. (**b**) Relative contribution of genes by the age at diagnosis of breast cancer women in 10-year-age groupings [3]

- Breast cancer onset at 45 years old or younger
- Triple-negative breast cancer (TNBC) onset at 60 years old or younger
- Onset of 2 or more primary breast cancers
- Family history of breast, ovarian, or pancreatic cancer up to third-degree
- Male breast cancer
- Having ovarian cancer, fallopian tube cancer, or peritoneal cancer

Fig. 2 *BRCA1/2* genetic testing criteria in Japanese breast cancer patients

3 Current Landscape of HBOC Care in Japan

Japan's universal health insurance system (since 1961) has facilitated access to specialized diagnostics and treatment. In 2018, *BRCA1/2* testing entered public coverage as a companion diagnostic for olaparib in metastatic/recurrent breast cancer; in 2020, coverage expanded to testing for HBOC diagnosis with defined eligibility criteria (Fig. 2). In response, relevant academic societies founded the Japan Organization of Hereditary Breast and Ovarian Cancer (JOHBOC), which has advanced education, guideline development, database construction, and workforce training—collectively accelerating nationwide implementation of HBOC care. Continued integration of public infrastructure and academic leadership is essential for a comprehensive, sustainable system.

4 Rationale for *BRCA1/2* Testing in Breast Clinics

Tertiary hospitals face mounting capacity constraints that hinder long-term postoperative follow-up. Currently, clinics focused on breast health, typically staffed by board-certified specialists, often serve as the initial point of medical contact for patients, providing comprehensive diagnostic services such as imaging and tissue sampling. In this context, offering HBOC-appropriate genetic testing at the initial diagnostic stage can inform surgical planning (e.g., breast conservation vs. risk-reducing procedures) and eligibility for perioperative PARP inhibitors, positioning BRCA status alongside pathology as a core determinant of management. Because *BRCA1/2* results typically require about 3 weeks, initiating counseling and testing only after referral to tertiary centers risks delaying treatment. Performing testing in clinics at the time of diagnosis can mitigate delays and also enable secondary screening of previously treated patients (particularly those managed before the April 2020 coverage expansion) who are now followed in community clinics.

To operationalize clinic-based testing, facilities should (i) notify regional health bureaus regarding compliance with testing standards; (ii) establish referral

Table 2 HBOC medical treatment introduction status

	E-learning seminars	Submission of facility notification	Number of genetic tests	Number of positive/VUS
Clinic A	Y	Y	17	2/0
Clinic B	Y	Y	39	0/0
Clinic C	Y	Y	84	5/3
Clinic D	Y	Y	0	0/0
Clinic E	Y	Y	0	0/0
Clinic F	Y	N	0	0/0
Clinic G	Y	Y	11	1/0

As of June 30, 2025

pathways with core hospitals and specialized genetics units for positive or VUS findings; and (iii) ensure staff complete accredited HBOC training (e.g., JOHBOC). In collaboration with multiple clinics in Tokyo, we have implemented these systems. As of 30 June 2025, many clinics have adopted the framework and are contributing to regionally integrated HBOC services (Table 2).

5 Operational Challenges of Clinic-Based Genetic Testing

Despite progress, several barriers remain. First, reimbursement lags can create sizable accounts receivable, posing financial risk for clinics. Second, the administrative load—facility notifications, inter-institutional agreements, and workforce training—can be substantial for small teams. Third, delivering timely genetic counseling immediately after a new cancer diagnosis is time- and psychology-intensive, complicating coordination with treatment discussions. Finally, employing full-time genetics-trained personnel is often impractical for private clinics due to recruitment and labor costs. Providing financial and institutional support, along with developing integrated-care models, may help address these gaps.

6 Conclusion

Japan has advanced HBOC care through early detection, personalized strategies, public insurance reforms, and coordinated academic efforts. Further strengthening clinic–tertiary center collaboration and ensuring timely, accurate delivery of genetic services are pivotal to a sustainable, equitable national HBOC system.

References

1. National Cancer Center Japan, Cancer Information Service. Accessed 2025.
2. Japanese Breast Cancer Society, Breast Cancer Registry. 2021. Accessed 2025.
3. Momozawa Y, et al. Germline pathogenic variants of 11 breast cancer genes in 7,051 Japanese patients and 11,241 controls. Nat Commun. 2018;9:4083.
4. Idogawa M, et al. The frequency and pathogenicity of BRCA1 and BRCA2 variants in the general Japanese population. J Hum Genet. 2024;69:225–30.

Regional Cooperation and Equalization in Clinical Practice for Hereditary Tumor Syndrome

Megumi Matsumoto, Aya Tanaka, Shoko Miura, Kiyonori Miura, and Keitaro Matsumoto

Abstract Significant regional disparities remain in the clinical management of hereditary tumors in Japan, particularly hereditary breast and ovarian cancer syndrome (HBOC). In recent years, insurance coverage for genetic testing, clinical surveillance, and risk-reducing surgery in cancer patients has expanded; however, a comprehensive, uniformly implemented system has not yet been established. For high-risk but unaffected individuals, substantial barriers to appropriate care persist, as surveillance methods such as contrast-enhanced breast MRI or preventive surgical interventions are available only as self-financed services. These challenges are even more pronounced in rural and island regions where access to specialists is limited.

In the Kyushu–Okinawa region, cross-prefectural cooperation has been actively developed to address these issues. In addition to the efforts of the Japanese Organization of Hereditary Breast and Ovarian Cancer (JOHBOC), the Kyushu Familial Cancer Network (KFCN), established in 2015, has played an essential role. This network connects 42 facilities across eight prefectures, enabling standardized data collection, shared resources, and improved patient accessibility. Furthermore,

M. Matsumoto (✉) · A. Tanaka
Division of Surgical Oncology, Department of Surgery, Nagasaki University Graduate School of Biomedical Sciences, Nagasaki, Japan

Breast and Endocrine Surgery, Department of Surgery, Nagasaki University Hospital, Nagasaki, Japan

Clinical Genomics Center, Nagasaki University Hospital, Nagasaki, Japan

S. Miura · K. Miura
Clinical Genomics Center, Nagasaki University Hospital, Nagasaki, Japan

Department of Obstetrics and Gynecology, Nagasaki University Graduate School of Biomedical Sciences, Nagasaki, Japan

K. Matsumoto
Division of Surgical Oncology, Department of Surgery, Nagasaki University Graduate School of Biomedical Sciences, Nagasaki, Japan

Breast and Endocrine Surgery, Department of Surgery, Nagasaki University Hospital, Nagasaki, Japan

M. Arai et al. (eds.), *Practical Guide to Hereditary Breast and Ovarian Cancer IV*,
https://doi.org/10.1007/978-981-95-6580-1_12

the joint educational activities and workforce development initiatives of KFCN and the Kyushu–Okinawa branch of the Regional Activation Committee of the Japanese Society for Genetic Counseling are laying the foundation for sustainable genetic medicine, extending beyond oncology to include reproductive medicine, nursing, and primary care.

This article highlights the progress and challenges observed in Nagasaki and the broader Kyushu–Okinawa region. By drawing on international guidelines, including those of the National Comprehensive Cancer Network (NCCN), the European Society for Medical Oncology (ESMO), and the American Society of Breast Surgeons (ASBrS), we identify areas requiring further development. These include the clinical implementation of multigene panel testing (MGPT), ethical considerations surrounding preimplantation genetic testing (PGT-M), and the need for multidisciplinary and cross-regional cooperation. Finally, we discuss future perspectives for establishing an equitable and patient-centered system of hereditary cancer care in Japan.

Keywords Hereditary tumor syndrome · Regional cooperation · HBOC · KFCN · Genetic counseling · Multigene panel testing

1 Introduction

Hereditary tumors present unique clinical and social challenges, as they affect not only patients themselves but also relatives who may share the same genetic predisposition. Among these, hereditary breast and ovarian cancer syndrome (HBOC) has been the most extensively studied and holds clinical importance. The identification of pathogenic variants in BRCA1/2 has enabled risk assessment, individualized surveillance, and preventive interventions for both patients and their families. Internationally, HBOC has become a model for integrating genetics into oncology, and its management has advanced markedly.

In Japan, HBOC is one of the few hereditary cancer syndromes for which certain genetic tests and related interventions are partially reimbursed by public health insurance. Since 2020, BRCA1/2 testing has been covered for breast cancer patients who meet specific criteria, representing a significant policy milestone. Nevertheless, the challenges remain. Insurance reimbursement is limited to selected breast cancer patients and all ovarian cancer patients, leaving predictive testing for unaffected relatives largely self-financed. Moreover, surveillance measures recommended by international guidelines—such as annual contrast-enhanced breast MRI beginning at age 25—are not uniformly reimbursed. Consequently, many individuals encounter significant financial and logistical barriers to appropriate preventive care. These disparities are further magnified in rural and island regions where access to specialists and MRI facilities is scarce.

International guidelines emphasize the importance of early and comprehensive intervention. The National Comprehensive Cancer Network (NCCN) [1] and the European Society for Medical Oncology (ESMO) [2] recommend annual MRI surveillance, risk-reducing mastectomy, and salpingo-oophorectomy as core strategies for BRCA mutation carriers. In 2019, the American Society of Breast Surgeons (ASBrS) issued a consensus statement recommending that all breast cancer patients have access to genetic testing, further underscoring the role of multigene panel testing (MGPT) [3]. MGPT allows simultaneous analysis of dozens to hundreds of cancer-related genes, providing a more comprehensive risk profile. However, this also raises new challenges, including the interpretation of variants of uncertain significance (VUS) [4], effective counseling of patients, and coordination of surveillance across multiple cancer types.

Japan faces unique systemic barriers in adapting these international standards. The scope of insurance coverage remains narrow, and preventive measures such as MRI or risk-reducing mastectomy are often excluded from reimbursement. Genetic counseling services are also unevenly distributed, being concentrated mainly in large academic centers. As a result, individuals living in regional or remote areas face substantial disparities in access. Even within a single prefecture, cooperation among relevant specialties—breast surgery, gynecology, urology, gastroenterology, and radiology—is sometimes insufficient, leading to fragmented care.

To address these inequities, regional and national networks have been established. The Japanese Organization of Hereditary Breast and Ovarian Cancer (JOHBOC), founded in 2016, has sought to reduce disparities through the accreditation of specialized facilities and professional training. In Kyushu, the Kyushu Familial Cancer Network (KFCN) was launched in 2015, pioneering cross-prefectural cooperation. KFCN links 42 facilities across eight prefectures in Kyushu and Okinawa, facilitating data sharing, standardization of care, and patient referral pathways. Beyond clinical cooperation, KFCN has emphasized education and workforce development and, in partnership with the Kyushu–Okinawa branch of the Regional Activation Committee of the Japanese Society for Genetic Counseling, has extended outreach to nurses, midwives, reproductive medicine professionals, and other allied health providers.

This article aims to situate the experiences of Nagasaki and the Kyushu–Okinawa region within the broader national and international context, clarifying both achievements and limitations. By examining how regional cooperation addresses systemic gaps, strengthens human resource capacity, and provides a model for future nationwide integration, we highlight critical issues that must be addressed to establish an equitable, sustainable, and patient-centered framework for hereditary cancer care in Japan.

2 Current Status of Hereditary Tumor Care in Nagasaki Prefecture

2.1 *Challenges in Breast Surveillance*

In Japan, surveillance for high-risk but unaffected individuals with a predisposition to breast or ovarian cancer remains outside the coverage of public health insurance. Consequently, patients must pay out of pocket for contrast-enhanced breast MRI or, in some cases, MRI-guided biopsy. International guidelines recommend annual contrast-enhanced breast MRI beginning at age 25–30 for women at high risk. However, because such examinations are self-financed in Japan, the financial burden creates a major barrier, potentially leading to delayed detection at an appropriate stage. Moreover, the interpretation of MRI requires advanced expertise, and cooperation with experienced radiologists is indispensable to ensure early and accurate diagnosis.

One of the key challenges in Nagasaki is the limited availability of such specialists. University hospitals play a central role, particularly in offering risk-reducing surgeries that fall outside the scope of insurance coverage. In contrast, many local hospitals and private clinics lack the equipment or trained personnel necessary to provide comprehensive surveillance. This uneven distribution of expertise has resulted in inconsistent quality of care within the prefecture.

2.2 *Breast Surveillance System and JOHBOC-Accredited Facilities*

In Nagasaki Prefecture, university hospitals are primarily responsible for procedures covered by insurance as well as risk-reducing surgeries provided as self-financed care. On the other hand, certain aspects of surveillance are delegated to nearby facilities. For example, St. Francis Hospital provides self-financed surveillance, while the Japanese Red Cross Nagasaki Genbaku Hospital offers MRI-guided biopsies conducted by experienced radiologists.

Nagasaki hosts both core and affiliated facilities accredited by the Japanese Organization of Hereditary Breast and Ovarian Cancer (JOHBOC), and the establishment of genetic counseling systems has been gradually advancing. Nevertheless, among the 27 institutions providing breast care in the prefecture, 11 remain unaffiliated with the JOHBOC network. Most of these are small clinics, and in practice, they generally refer patients to Nagasaki University Hospital when genetic testing is required. Furthermore, only a limited number of facilities can perform risk-reducing mastectomy (RRM), leaving high-risk patients with insufficient access to surgical preventive options. This situation highlights the urgent need to further expand facilities and human resources capable of providing specialized preventive care.

2.3 *Insufficient Cooperation with Other Clinical Departments*

Another significant challenge in Nagasaki is the lack of structured cooperation with departments that treat HBOC-related cancers, such as prostate and pancreatic cancer. With the increasing use of multigene panel testing (MGPT), more carriers at risk for multiple hereditary tumors are expected to be identified. Without a robust interdisciplinary framework, however, the delivery of appropriate surveillance and preventive interventions may become inconsistent. Such fragmented care risks undermining the benefits of advanced genetic testing and may leave patients without clear follow-up strategies.

Therefore, establishing strong interdisciplinary networks—including oncology, urology, gastroenterology, gynecology, and radiology—is essential for the effective implementation of MGPT-based care in Nagasaki. Such an integrated system would not only enhance clinical practice but also contribute to reducing disparities in access to specialized care across the prefecture.

3 Wide-Area Cooperation in the Kyushu–Okinawa Region

3.1 *Establishment and Activities of the Kyushu Familial Cancer Network (KFCN)*

The Kyushu Familial Cancer Network (KFCN) was established in 2015 with the goal of reducing regional disparities in hereditary tumor care through cross-prefectural cooperation. As of 2025, the network includes 42 facilities across eight prefectures, ranging from academic institutions to community hospitals. Its activities span information sharing, surveys of diagnostic and therapeutic systems, educational initiatives targeting healthcare professionals, and the development and dissemination of standardized consent forms. By creating these frameworks, KFCN has succeeded in fostering cooperation that transcends both institutional and prefectural boundaries.

Importantly, KFCN has provided a valuable forum for professional exchange. Regular forums bring together specialists from diverse disciplines—including oncology, genetics, gynecology, and nursing—thereby forming an integrated platform to advance hereditary tumor medicine. Notably, the network operates on a voluntary basis without collecting participation fees yet has managed to sustain a wide range of activities since its inception.

3.2 Data Collection and Information Sharing

Since its establishment, KFCN has conducted multiple questionnaire surveys of participating institutions to assess the state of hereditary tumor care. These surveys have documented the availability of genetic counseling, surveillance, and risk-reducing surgery for conditions such as HBOC, Lynch syndrome, familial adenomatous polyposis (FAP), and multiple endocrine neoplasia (MEN). The aggregated data have been used to identify gaps in service provision and to inform strategic planning across the region.

Furthermore, KFCN maintains a publicly accessible website that lists participating institutions. The website not only provides the names of the facilities but also specifies the scope of genetic services available at each site, including genetic counseling, surveillance, and preventive surgery. This system allows patients and families to directly identify and contact appropriate facilities, thereby enhancing transparency and facilitating timely access to care. Such open disclosure is rare in Japan's medical context and represents a significant step toward more patient-centered care.

3.3 Strengths and Challenges of Wide-Area Cooperation

The wide-area approach adopted in Kyushu and Okinawa demonstrates the potential of regional networks to reduce disparities. By pooling resources and expertise, KFCN has enabled facilities with limited capacity to refer patients more efficiently and to participate in standardized educational programs. However, sustaining such a network requires the continuous allocation of financial and human resources. As genetic medicine expands and more institutions participate, maintaining the administration of the network—including the management of its secretariat, forums, surveys, and data analysis—has become increasingly difficult.

Nevertheless, KFCN serves as an important model for Japan, showing how regional cooperation can go beyond isolated institutional initiatives to establish coordinated systems of care. Looking ahead, the network hopes not only to strengthen cooperation within Kyushu and Okinawa but also to connect with other regional networks across the country, ultimately aspiring to create a nationwide system that links all of Japan.

4 Human Resource Development and Genetic Medicine Network

4.1 Development of Professionals

The advancement of hereditary tumor care requires not only cooperation between institutions but also the systematic training of professionals across diverse disciplines. In the Kyushu–Okinawa region, this effort has been promoted through the activities of the Kyushu Familial Cancer Network (KFCN). In parallel, the Regional Activation Committee of the Japanese Society for Genetic Counseling and the Kyushu–Yamaguchi CGC Network have also undertaken similar initiatives. Collectively, these activities emphasize education and awareness not only for physicians but also for nurses, midwives, reproductive medicine specialists, certified genetic counselors, and other healthcare professionals.

Regular seminars, workshops, and support programs for individuals and families affected by hereditary tumors provide valuable opportunities for young healthcare providers to gain expertise in genetic medicine. In these programs, participants propose current challenges, which are then addressed through lectures delivered by experts most familiar with the issue, followed by interactive workshops. Importantly, these initiatives are not limited to oncology but have also extended to reproductive and perinatal medicine, reflecting the broad relevance of genetics across the continuum of care.

Training a diverse workforce is critical to ensure that hereditary tumor care—and genetic medicine more broadly—is not confined to a small number of academic centers. Strengthening the capacity of regional institutions allows patients in rural and remote areas to access essential medical services, thereby reducing disparities in healthcare delivery.

4.2 The Need for Cooperation Beyond Oncology

Although hereditary tumor syndromes such as HBOC currently serve as the focal point of these initiatives, the scope of genetic medicine is rapidly expanding. Advances in genomic technologies now enable the identification of genetic predispositions not only for cancer but also for cardiovascular, neurological, and metabolic disorders. Therefore, future regional networks must broaden their focus beyond oncology and establish cooperative frameworks with specialists in multiple clinical fields.

This expansion of scope also highlights the necessity of robust communication platforms that connect professionals and institutions. By sharing data, clinical experiences, and educational resources, networks such as KFCN, together with allied initiatives, can serve as incubators for cross-disciplinary innovation. Moreover, incorporating patient-support activities into training programs equips healthcare providers with the skills needed to address the complex medical, ethical, and psychosocial needs of individuals and families living with genetic risk.

Ultimately, fostering a multidisciplinary and geographically diverse workforce is indispensable for building a sustainable and equitable system of genetic medicine. Such a system must be able to adapt to new technologies, confront emerging ethical challenges, and provide comprehensive support for patients throughout their life course.

5 Discussion

The future of hereditary tumor care in Japan is expected to present a variety of challenges. Among the most significant is the introduction of multigene panel testing (MGPT). Even in hereditary breast cancer alone, multiple germline genes have been identified as contributors [4]. MGPT enables the simultaneous analysis of dozens to hundreds of genes, offering great potential for risk assessment and early detection across a wide range of cancers. At the same time, however, it raises new challenges, including the interpretation of variants of uncertain significance (VUS), the necessity of comprehensive genetic counseling before and after testing, and the establishment of multidisciplinary frameworks to coordinate surveillance and preventive strategies across different cancer types [5].

Another important issue is preimplantation genetic testing for monogenic disorders (PGT-M), which considers the transmission of pathogenic variants to the next generation. In Japan, PGT-M is regulated primarily under an application system managed by the Japan Society of Obstetrics and Gynecology [6]. However, this system involves complex challenges, including ethical concerns, social implications, and the perspectives of affected individuals [7]. As genetic technologies continue to advance, striking a balance between patient autonomy, reproductive choice, and societal values will remain a crucial topic of discussion.

Addressing these challenges requires the establishment of both regional and nationwide collaborative systems. Networks such as the Kyushu Familial Cancer Network (KFCN) and the Regional Activation Committee of the Japanese Society for Genetic Counseling provide successful examples of reducing disparities, promoting professional education, and expanding access to genetic services. The key to sustaining such initiatives lies in building "visible relationships" that foster trust and cooperation across prefectures, specialties, and institutions.

Furthermore, Japan must align its strategies with international standards while adapting them to its unique healthcare system and cultural context. Guidelines from organizations such as the National Comprehensive Cancer Network (NCCN) [1] and the European Society for Medical Oncology (ESMO) [2] emphasize early and proactive management. However, in Japan, insurance limitations and regional disparities hinder their full implementation [8, 9]. Bridging these gaps will require policy reform, expanded insurance coverage, and the integration of telemedicine and digital platforms to ensure equitable access across all regions, including rural and island communities.

Ultimately, this discussion demonstrates that the future of hereditary cancer care in Japan depends on both technological innovation and the strengthening of human and institutional networks. By expanding the scope of cooperation, investing in workforce development, and embedding ethical perspectives into clinical practice, Japan can progress toward a more equitable, sustainable, and patient-centered model of hereditary cancer management.

6 Conclusion

Regional cooperation in hereditary cancer care in Nagasaki and the Kyushu–Okinawa region remains a work in progress but has been steadily advancing. These initiatives demonstrate that disparities across prefectures can be reduced through cooperative frameworks, shared expertise, and cross-institutional referral systems. Moving forward, it will be essential to further expand human resource development, strengthen cooperation across multiple clinical disciplines, and build an integrated framework of genetic medicine that is both comprehensive and patient-centered. Ultimately, the establishment of such a system will be critical for achieving equity and sustainability in hereditary tumor management throughout Japan.

Acknowledgements The author would like to express sincere gratitude to all members of the Kyushu Familial Cancer Network (KFCN) and to the Kyushu–Okinawa branch of the Regional Activation Committee of the Japanese Society for Genetic Counseling for their invaluable contributions and continued cooperation in advancing hereditary cancer care. We would like to thank Editage (www.editage.jp) for English language editing.

Conflicts of Interest (COI) The author declares no conflicts of interest related to this manuscript.

References

1. National Comprehensive Cancer Network. NCCN Clinical Practice Guidelines in Oncology. Genetic/familial high-risk assessment: breast, ovarian, pancreatic, and prostate Version 1.2026. https://www.nccn.org/professionals/physician_gls/pdf/genetics_bopp.pdf. Access 2025/08/31.
2. Sessa C, Balmaña J, Bober SL, Cardoso MJ, Colombo N, Curigliano G, Domchek SM, Evans DG, Fischerova D, Harbeck N, Kuhl C, Lemley B, Levy-Lahad E, Lambertini M, Ledermann JA, Loibl S, Phillips KA, Paluch-Shimon S, ESMO Guidelines Committee. Electronic address: clinicalguidelines@esmo.org. Risk reduction and screening of cancer in hereditary breast-ovarian cancer syndromes: ESMO clinical practice guideline. Ann Oncol. 2023;34(1):33–47. https://doi.org/10.1016/j.annonc.2022.10.004. Epub 2022 Oct 25. PMID: 36307055
3. Manahan ER, Kuerer HM, Sebastian M, Hughes KS, Boughey JC, Euhus DM, Boolbol SK, Taylor WA. Consensus guidelines on genetic` testing for hereditary breast cancer from the American Society of Breast Surgeons. Ann Surg Oncol. 2019;26(10):3025–31. https://doi.org/10.1245/s10434-019-07549-8. Epub 2019 Jul 24. PMID: 31342359; PMCID: PMC6733830
4. Momozawa Y, Iwasaki Y, Parsons MT, Kamatani Y, Takahashi A, Tamura C, Katagiri T, Yoshida T, Nakamura S, Sugano K, Miki Y, Hirata M, Matsuda K, Spurdle AB,

Kubo M. Germline pathogenic variants of 11 breast cancer genes in 7,051 Japanese patients and 11,241 controls. Nat Commun. 2018;9(1):4083. https://doi.org/10.1038/s41467-018-06581-8. PMID: 30287823; PMCID: PMC6172276
5. Kurian AW, Ward KC, Hamilton AS, Deapen DM, Abrahamse P, Bondarenko I, Li Y, Hawley ST, Morrow M, Jagsi R, Katz SJ. Uptake, results, and outcomes of germline multiple-gene sequencing after diagnosis of breast cancer. JAMA Oncol. 2018;4(8):1066–72. https://doi.org/10.1001/jamaoncol.2018.0644. PMID: 29801090; PMCID: PMC6143044
6. Japan Society of Obstetrics and Gynecology. https://www.jsog.or.jp/medical/868/. Access 2025/08/31.
7. Calosci D, Passaglia L, Gabbiato I, Cartisano F, Affuso R, Sorrentino U, Zuccarello D. Public awareness and acceptability of PGT-M in cancer predisposition syndromes. Genes (Basel). 2023;14(11):2069. https://doi.org/10.3390/genes14112069. PMID: 38003012; PMCID: PMC10671058
8. Ohsumi S, Nakamura S, Miyata H, Watanabe C, Den H, Arai M. Risk-reducing mastectomy for women with hereditary breast and ovarian cancer (HBOC): analytical results of data from the Japanese organization of HBOC. Jpn J Clin Oncol. 2022;52(11):1265–9. https://doi.org/10.1093/jjco/hyac120. PMID: 35905458
9. Matsumoto M, Den H, Miura S, Harada A, Nomura H, Arai M, Kumamaru H, Nakamura S, Sekine M, Miura K. The impact of public insurance on RRSO for HBOC in Japan: a nationwide data study. J Hum Genet. 2025;70(8):421–6. https://doi.org/10.1038/s10038-025-01326-0. Epub 2025 May 21. PMID: 40399479; PMCID: PMC12289518

Present Status and Issue of Cooperation of HBOC Clinical Practice in Niigata Prefecture

Koji Nishino

1 Introduction

Niigata Prefecture is a heavy snowfall area facing the Sea of Japan, with a population of approximately 2.3 million. It spans about 330 km in length and is the fifth largest prefecture in Japan (Fig. 1). With approximately 1300 new cases of breast cancer and 100 new cases of ovarian cancer occurring annually, it is estimated that approximately 100 new cases of HBOC occur overall. Niigata Prefecture is vast and includes a remote island (Sado Island), making the need for collaboration and self-sufficiency within the prefecture itself regarding HBOC management greater than in other regions..

2 Launch of the Department of Familial and Hereditary Oncology at Niigata University

The Department of Familial and Hereditary Oncology was established at Niigata University with a donation from Niigata Prefecture in November 2016, and constructed a collaborative framework between Niigata Prefecture and Niigata University for HBOC management.

K. Nishino (✉)
Department of Gynecologic Oncology, Niigata Cancer Center Hospital, Niigata, Japan

Department of Familial and Hereditary Oncology (Obstetrics and Gynecology), Niigata University Graduate School of Medical and Dental Sciences, Niigata, Japan
e-mail: knishino@med.niigata-u.ac.jp

M. Arai et al. (eds.), *Practical Guide to Hereditary Breast and Ovarian Cancer IV*,
https://doi.org/10.1007/978-981-95-6580-1_13

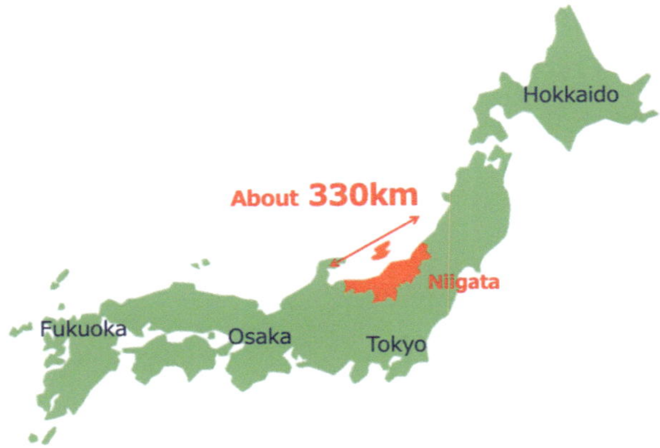

Fig. 1 Niigata Prefecture in Japan. Niigata Prefecture is a heavy snowfall area facing the Sea of Japan, with a population of approximately 2.3 million. It spans about 330 km in length and is the fifth largest prefecture in Japan

3 Establishment and Initiation of RRSO Within Niigata Prefecture

One of the goals of HBOC management is to provide risk-reducing surgery for at-risk individuals who have pathogenic germline variants of *BRCA1/2*. Especially, risk-reducing salpingo-oophorectomy (RRSO) holds significant importance as the only recommended method for ovarian cancer prevention in HBOC. Since establishing the Department of Familial and Hereditary Oncology, we have developed a system for performing RRSO in Niigata. Following Japanese insurance approval of RRSO in April 2020, we have received referrals from both within and outside the Niigata prefecture, and not only from gynecologists but also from breast surgeons, performing over 40 RRSOs by the end of October 2023. In particular, breast surgery (risk-reducing mastectomy or breast cancer surgery) is performed concurrently with RRSO in approximately half of all cases, which can be attributed to the success of collaboration within our facility.

4 Issues in HBOC Management in Niigata Prefecture

1. *Regional Disparities*

   Within Niigata Prefecture, the number of medical hospitals differs between urban and countryside areas, and this disparity was also reflected in the differences in the actual performed number of BRACAnalysis.
2. *Centralization and Division of Roles*

   There are two JOHBOC-certified facilities within Niigata prefecture, both located in close proximity to each other in central Niigata City. Initially, our HBOC-management plan was to divide the roles: providing genetic counseling/testing, performing risk-reducing surgery at certified facilities (Central Niigata city), while local facilities would handle identifying at-risk individuals and conducting surveillance. However, patient transfers within the Niigata prefecture posed a significant burden actually, and certified facilities saw a marked increase in HBOC cases, leading us to conclude that there were limits to the division of roles they could play within the Niigata prefecture. In other words, there appears to be a need to establish a certain level of HBOC management locally.

3. *Ensuring the Quality of Genetic Management*

   JOHBOC-certified facilities employ board-certified specialists (gynecologists, breast surgeons, genetic counselors, and genetic specialists) who provide high-quality HBOC care, including conducting educational training on HBOC and maintaining family registries for HBOC patients. To receive high-quality HBOC care in Niigata, it may be advisable for patients to visit JOHBOC-certified facilities. However, this involves significant burdens, including patient transportation for long distance actually. Therefore, improving and maintaining the quality of genetic medicine at local facilities is crucial.

5 Conclusion

This chapter introduced collaborative efforts for HBOC management in Niigata Prefecture.

A Familial and Hereditary Oncology Department was established at Niigata University through a donation from Niigata Prefecture. The effectiveness of collaboration in and outside the prefecture is demonstrated by the achievement of establishing an RRSO implementation system and receiving referrals from both in and outside the prefecture.

However, regional disparities exist within Niigata. While it is necessary to complete genetic medical care locally, this also requires ensuring the quality of both practice and research. Therefore, it is desirable to effectively utilize the JOHBOC-facility certification system.

Equalization of Care and Regional Cooperation in Clinical Practice for Hereditary Tumors Using Public Data

Yuko Minoura

Abstract The fourth Basic Plan to Promote Cancer Control Programs states: "In addition to equalizing, promote consolidation per the specific conditions present in each region through role sharing and collaboration between designated cancer care hospitals." Against this policy background, the present study examined how *BRCA1/2* genetic testing and the treatment for hereditary breast and ovarian cancer (HBOC), as a representative model for hereditary tumor management in Japan, should be equalized and consolidated within the framework of public health insurance practices.

Keywords Equalization and consolidation · Public health insurance · Designated cancer care hospitals

1 Introduction

The introduction of public health insurance coverage to reimburse *BRCA1/2* genetic testing for the diagnosis of hereditary breast and ovarian cancer (HBOC) in April 2020 signified substantial advancements in the field of gene oncology in Japan. This policy change has integrated *BRCA1/2* genetic testing into routine medical care. Concurrently, the adoption of comprehensive genomic profiling for advanced and metastatic cancers further expanded physician awareness of hereditary tumors.

Approximately 110,000 new breast cancer cases, including carcinoma in situ, are diagnosed annually in Japan [7]. Among these, an estimated 4–5% of individuals carry pathogenic variants in their germline *BRCA1/2* genes [6], corresponding to around 5000 breast cancer cases attributable to HBOC each year. Because no

Y. Minoura (✉)
Department of Clinical Genetics Oncology, The Cancer Institute Hospital of JFCR, Tokyo, Japan
e-mail: yuko.minoura@jfcr.or.jp

M. Arai et al. (eds.), *Practical Guide to Hereditary Breast and Ovarian Cancer IV*, https://doi.org/10.1007/978-981-95-6580-1_14

significant regional disparities exist among patients with breast cancer or HBOC, equitable nationwide access to HBOC treatment is essential.

In its 4th Basic Plan to Promote Cancer Control Programs [2], the Ministry of Health, Labor, and Welfare stated, "In addition to equalizing, promote consolidation per the specific conditions present in each region through role sharing and collaboration between designated cancer care hospitals." Declines in regional populations underscore the increasing need to consider which medical services should be equalized nationwide and which should be consolidated regionally.

This chapter examined the treatment of HBOC under health insurance coverage in Japan by analyzing the current situation and describes approaches for equalizing and consolidating the management of hereditary tumors.

2 Methods

I obtained a list of medical institutions that submitted facility notification forms from each Regional Bureau of Health and Welfare website. I then confirmed the status of facility notification forms related to HBOC treatment as of June 1, 2025, including *BRCA1/2* genetic testing (GT), genetic counseling (GC) with additional fee, and surgeries listed in Section 19 of Chapter 2, Part 10 of the Medical Fee Score Table ("resection of uterine adnexal tumors in patients with HBOC, risk-reducing salpingo-oophorectomy, RRSO" and "mastectomy, limited to procedures performed in patients with HBOC, risk-reducing mastectomy, RRM").

Population data by sex and age (in 5-year intervals) for each prefecture as of October 1, 2024, were obtained from the Statistics Bureau, Ministry of Internal Affairs and Communications website. Data on the area of each prefecture, as of April 1, 2025, were obtained from the Geospatial Information Authority of Japan, Ministry of Land, Infrastructure, Transport, and Tourism websites. Using these data, I analyzed the implementation status of HBOC treatment in each prefecture, focusing on the female population aged ≥15 years, as well as the implementation status per 1000 km^2. Using these data, we generated maps with QGIS (QGIS Development Team, 2025 [9]), an open-source geographic information system.

For reference, *BRCA1/2* genetic testing data (based on blood samples) were extracted from the National Database (NDB) 2021 claims information, and the 2021 incidence rate of breast cancer (including carcinoma in situ) by prefecture was extracted from the National Cancer Registry.

3 Results

Of the 1416 medical institutions nationwide able to perform GT, 513 (36.2%) could also perform GC in-house. Among GT-performing facilities, 284 (20.1%) and 248 (17.5%) reported performing RRSO and RRM, respectively.

After GT, the proportion of medical institutions able to provide GC in-house (GT + GC) varied markedly by prefecture. Values ranged from 71.4% (5/7) in the prefecture with the highest value and 50.0% (11/22, 20/40) in the second-highest prefecture to 18.2% (4/22) in the second-lowest prefecture and 5.9% (1/17) in the lowest prefecture (interquartile range [IQR]: 17.6%). Among GT-performing facilities, 50.0% (4/8) in the highest prefecture and 42.9% (3/7) in the second-highest prefecture could perform RRSO, whereas in six prefectures, only a single facility offered RRSO. The top two prefectures for RRM were the same as those for RRSO, whereas five prefectures had only one RRM-capable facility and one prefecture had none.

Nationwide, RRSO-capable facilities numbered 0.50 per 100,000 females aged ≥15 years, with substantial prefectural variation: 1.36 in the highest prefecture, 1.01 in the second-highest prefecture, and 0.13 in the lowest two prefectures (IQR: 0.347). RRM-capable facilities accounted for 0.44 per 100,000 females aged ≥15 years nationwide, ranging from 1.36 to 0.13 (IQR: 0.339), excluding the prefecture lacking facilities capable of implementing (Fig. 1).

The number of RRSO facilities per 1000 km^2 of prefectural area was 0.75 nationwide, 15.91 in the highest prefecture, 12.07 in the second-highest prefecture, and 0.13 in the lowest three prefectures (IQR: 0.713). Similarly, the number of RRM facilities was 0.66 nationwide, 14.55 in the highest prefecture, 12.07 in the second-highest prefecture, and 0.08 in the lowest prefecture (IQR: 0.758) (Fig. 2).

According to the government's classification of designated cancer care hospitals, all prefectural designated cancer care hospitals could implement GT + GC and RRSO and 94.1% (48/51) could implement RRM. The feasibility at regional designated cancer care hospitals was as follows: GT, 96.6% (340/352); GT + GC, 75.3% (265/352); RRSO, 48.6% (171/352); and RRM, 41.5% (146/352). In contrast, at regional cancer care hospitals, GT was feasible in 83.1% (49/59) of facilities, GT + GC in 8.5% (5/59), RRSO in 1.7% (1/59), and RRM in 0.0% (0/59) (Fig. 3).

For reference, in 2021, *BRCA1/2* genetic tests using blood samples were performed in 22.3% of patients with breast cancer (note: the number of patients who underwent this genetic test including those with other cancer types). Prefectural rates ranged from 32.2% in the highest prefecture (A) and 31.8% in the second-highest prefecture (B) to 6.2% in the second-lowest prefecture (C) and 4.3% in the lowest prefecture (D) (IQR: 9.2%). *BRCA1/2* genetic testing is often conducted for confirmation in younger patients with breast cancer. The proportions of tested patients aged 15–44 years diagnosed with breast cancer did not differ significantly among prefectures, at 10.3% in A, 11.4% in B, 11.9% in C, and 8.8% in D.

4 Discussion

Five years have passed since *BRCA1/2* genetic testing for HBOC diagnosis became covered by public health insurance. Although treatment for HBOC is increasingly recognized as standard practice, the results of this survey revealed substantial

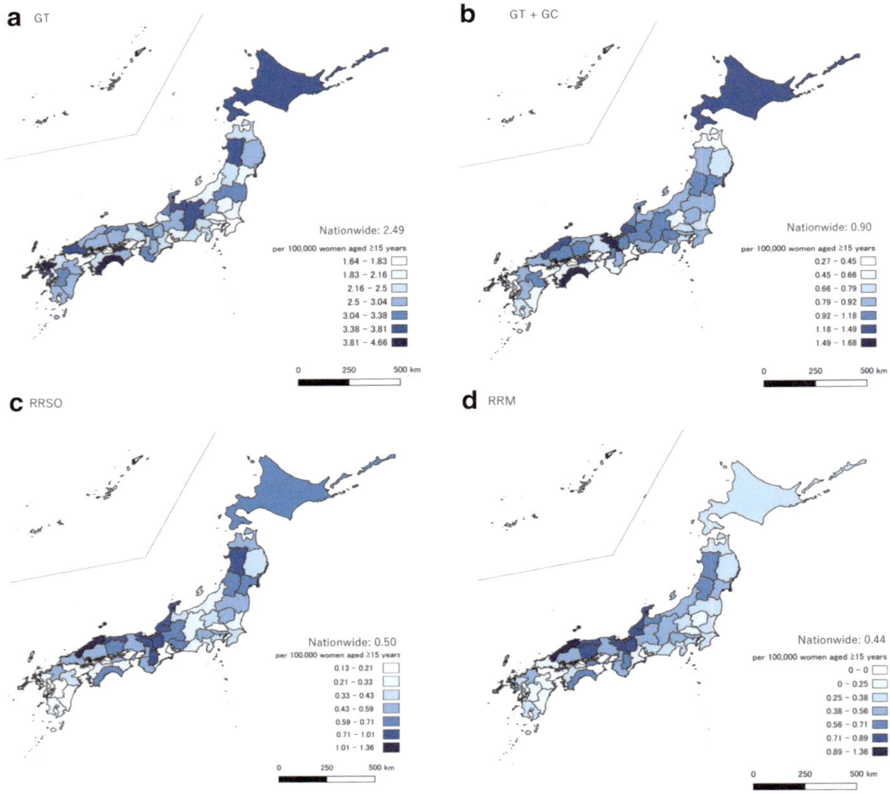

Fig. 1 Number of facilities capable of performing each medical procedure per 100,000 women aged ≥15 years in each prefecture. (**a**) GT-capable facilities. (**b**) GT + GC-capable facilities. (**c**) RRSO-capable facilities. (**d**) RRM-capable facilities. Darker hues indicate a higher prevalence. Base map data from the Geospatial Information Authority of Japan (GSI). GT, genetic testing; GC, genetic counseling; RRSO, risk-reducing salpingo-oophorectomy; RRM, risk-reducing mastectomy

variation in the availability of each medical procedure across prefectures. Nationwide, among facilities capable of performing GT, only approximately 35% could perform GC, and only around 20% could perform risk-reducing surgery.

The number of facilities capable of performing each medical procedure per population and area differed significantly among prefectures. Differences in population composition, traffic infrastructure, hospital size, and number of clinics suggest that these survey figures alone are insufficient to fully reflect the actual situation in each region. Nevertheless, given the marked regional differences in the ratio of patients with breast cancer to *BRCA1/2* genetic testing, disparities in HBOC treatment among prefectures are likely, although this remains an inference because *BRCA1/2* testing includes companion diagnostics and testing in patients without breast cancer.

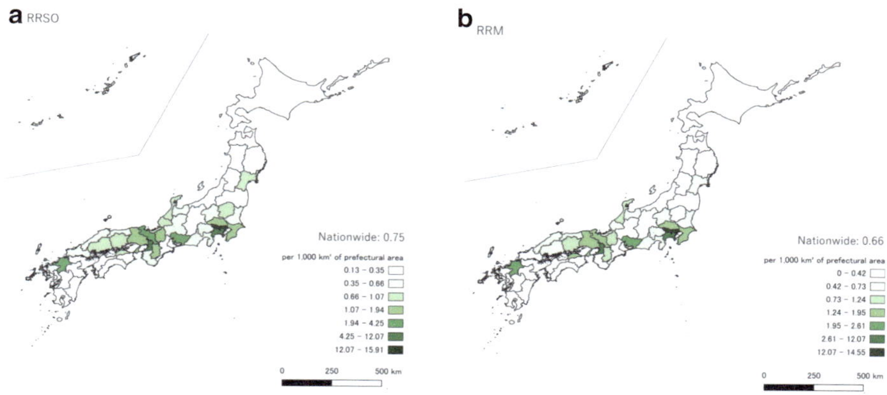

Fig. 2 Number of facilities capable of performing each medical procedure per 1000 km² of prefectural area. Darker hues indicate a higher prevalence. Base map data from the Geospatial Information Authority of Japan (GSI). (**a**) RRSO-capable facilities, (**b**) RRM-capable facilities. RRSO: risk-reducing salpingo-oophorectomy, RRM: risk-reducing mastectomy

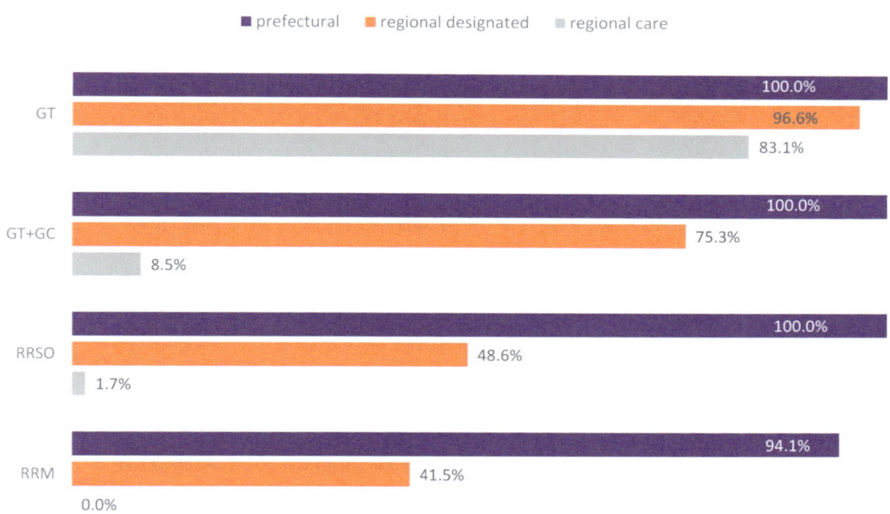

Fig. 3 Proportions of facilities capable of performing each medical procedure according to the designated cancer care hospital classification. Prefectural: prefectural designated cancer care hospitals ($n = 51$); regional designated: regional designated cancer care hospitals ($n = 352$); regional care: regional cancer care hospitals ($n = 59$)

Analysis by type of designated cancer care hospital revealed that prefectural designated cancer care hospitals, which exist in at least one location per prefecture and serve as central hubs for cancer care, generally provide treatment for HBOC, including risk-reducing surgery, in almost all prefectures. At regional-designated cancer care hospitals established in each cancer care area, GT + GC was feasible in 75% of the hospitals, while risk-reducing surgery was feasible in slightly fewer than half. Regional cancer care hospitals that collaborate with these facilities can perform GT but typically rely on their partner hospitals for other HBOC treatments.

HBOC affects an estimated 1 in 300–500 individuals globally [5, 6, 11], making it relatively common. Once diagnosed, patient prognosis can be improved through drug selection [10], risk-reducing surgery [1], and magnetic resonance imaging (MRI)-based surveillance [4]. Genetic testing of relatives is also recommended [8]. Guidelines advise offering genetic testing information to eligible patients with breast or ovarian cancer under public health insurance coverage [3], with respect to the patient's decision. Therefore, a low implementation rate does not necessarily indicate that information is not being provided; however, low implementation generally correlates with fewer HBOC diagnoses. Additionally, referral rates from facilities unable to perform GC cannot be determined from these data. Matters other than treatment will likely be put on hold during cancer treatment because treatment is the top priority. When GT is performed at a clinic, patients are typically referred to collaborating hospitals for standard treatments such as surgery and chemotherapy. Therefore, even a positive GT result is likely to lead to GC or risk-reducing surgery. However, regional cancer care hospitals often perform standard treatments. Therefore, the fact that only 8.5% of hospitals have the capacity to perform GC, with many lacking facilities to perform risk-reducing surgery, cannot be ruled out as a factor influencing HBOC treatment options.

Risk-reducing surgery is not recommended for all HBOC patients with cancer [3]. Because these surgeries are less urgent than cancer treatment, not all hospitals providing cancer care need to perform this procedure. Nevertheless, each prefecture should have at least one facility capable of performing risk-reducing surgery for HBOC, reflecting the concentration of advanced cancer treatments, except for pediatric and rare cancers, at the prefectural level. As of June 2025, RRM cannot be performed in one prefecture, highlighting the need for a system to facilitate its implementation.

In summary, it is important that genetic testing be available for HBOC diagnosis regardless of where the patient is diagnosed with cancer, and equal access to genetic counseling is important to avoid influencing treatment decisions. Conversely, risk-reducing surgery and surveillance require specialized expertise, supporting the consolidation of these procedures. Moreover, developing referral and cooperation systems tailored to the specific needs of each region is crucial.

5 Conclusion

This study examined the equalization and consolidation of medical care for HBOC, currently implemented as a pioneering treatment for hereditary tumors in Japan. With advances in personalized medicine, public health insurance may cover other hereditary tumor syndromes in the future. Designing systems that ensure both equalization and consolidation will be essential.

Competing Interests The author declares no conflicts of interest relevant to the contents of this chapter.

References

1. Domchek SM, Friebel TM, Singer CF, et al. Association of Risk-Reducing Surgery in BRCA1 or BRCA2 mutation carriers with cancer risk and mortality. JAMA. 2010;304:967–75. https://doi.org/10.1001/jama.2010.1237.
2. Foundation for Promotion of Cancer Research. Cancer_statistics_2024. 2024. https://ganjoho.jp/public/qa_links/report/statistics/pdf/cancer_statistics_2024_pre_E.pdf. Accessed 23 Aug 2025.
3. Japanese Organization of Hereditary Breast and Ovarian Cancer. Guideline for Diagnosis and Treatment of Hereditary Breast and Ovarian Cancer 2024. In: Guideline for Diagnosis and Treatment of Hereditary Breast and Ovarian Cancer 2024. 2024. https://johboc.jp/guidebook_2024. Accessed 24 Aug 2025.
4. Lubinski J, Kotsopoulos J, Moller P, et al. MRI surveillance and breast cancer mortality in women with *BRCA1* and *BRCA2* sequence variations. JAMA Oncol. 2024; https://doi.org/10.1001/jamaoncol.2023.6944.
5. Momozawa Y, Iwasaki Y, Hirata M, et al. Germline pathogenic variants in 7636 Japanese patients with prostate cancer and 12 366 controls. JNCI J Natl Cancer Inst. 2020;112:369–76. https://doi.org/10.1093/jnci/djz124.
6. Momozawa Y, Iwasaki Y, Parsons MT, et al. Germline pathogenic variants of 11 breast cancer genes in 7,051 Japanese patients and 11,241 controls. Nat Commun. 2018;9:4083. https://doi.org/10.1038/s41467-018-06581-8.
7. National Cancer Center. Cancer statistics in Japan; table download:[National Cancer Center cancer statistics]. In: National Cancer Center cancer statistics. 2025. https://ganjoho.jp/reg_stat/statistics/data/dl/en.html. Accessed 24 Aug 2025.
8. National Comprehensive Cancer Network.Genetic/familial high-risk assessment: breast, ovarian, pancreatic, and prostate. 2025.
9. QGIS Development Team. QGIS Geographic Information System. Open Source Geospatial Foundation; 2025. Available from: https://qgis.org.
10. Robson ME, Tung N, Conte P, et al. OlympiAD final overall survival and tolerability results: Olaparib versus chemotherapy treatment of physician's choice in patients with a germline BRCA mutation and HER2-negative metastatic breast cancer. Ann Oncol. 2019;30:558–66. https://doi.org/10.1093/annonc/mdz012.
11. Usui Y, Iwasaki Y, Matsuo K, et al. Association between germline pathogenic variants in cancer-predisposing genes and lymphoma risk. Cancer Sci. 2022;113:3972–9. https://doi.org/10.1111/cas.15522.

Expanding Opportunities and Evolving Challenges in the Genetic Diagnosis and Genetic Counseling of Hereditary Tumors in Japan

Akihiro Sakurai

Abstract The genetic diagnosis and counseling of hereditary cancer syndromes have shifted from specialized centers to become an essential part of oncology practice. Advances in sequencing and companion diagnostics have increased testing opportunities, with *BRCA1/2* at the forefront due to its dual role in preventing and treating cancer with PARP inhibitors. In Japan, these developments coincide with a universal insurance system that regulates genetic testing through "notified facilities."

Unlike most single-gene tests under code D006-4, which require ordering by notified facilities, *BRCA* testing (D006-18) can be initiated by non-notified hospitals if they provide genetic counselling in collaboration with a notified facility. While this framework is intended to safeguard quality, it has created barriers. Only around 25% of *BRCA* PV-positive patients were referred to notified facilities for counseling and cascade testing. Reasons include physician workload, patient reluctance, and limited referral pathways. Internationally, cascade testing uptake rarely exceeds 40%, reflecting the difficulty of disclosing hereditary risk to relatives.

Japan reimburses remote genetic counseling, but only for rare diseases, excluding hereditary breast and ovarian cancer (HBOC). To address this gap, we established a self-funded remote counseling model ("Dr-to-Patient-with-Dr"), linking local hospitals with genetics specialists. This system reduces patient travel burden and supports local clinicians but raises concerns about cost, technical feasibility, and counseling depth.

This proceeding reviews Japanese and global experiences, emphasizing systemic and psychosocial barriers. Key lessons include the need to integrate genetic diagnosis into oncology, provide family-centered psychosocial support, and expand innovative models such as remote counseling to improve access.

Keywords Hereditary cancer · *BRCA* testing · Genetic counseling · Cascade testing · Remote counseling

---

A. Sakurai (✉)
Department of Clinical Genomics, Division of Genomic and Preventive Medicine, Sapporo Medical University School of Medicine, Chuo-ku, Sapporo, Japan

M. Arai et al. (eds.), *Practical Guide to Hereditary Breast and Ovarian Cancer IV*,
https://doi.org/10.1007/978-981-95-6580-1_15

1 Introduction

The landscape of hereditary cancer diagnosis has changed profoundly over the past two decades. Once considered the domain of specialized centers with expertise in rare familial cancer syndromes, the field has now entered mainstream oncology. Advances in molecular biology, next-generation sequencing (NGS), and the integration of companion diagnostics into standard cancer care have all contributed to this shift. At the same time, the availability of preventive strategies such as prophylactic surgery and enhanced surveillance has underscored the clinical utility of hereditary cancer diagnosis.

Hereditary breast and ovarian cancer (HBOC), caused by germline pathogenic variants in *BRCA1* or *BRCA2*, has become the most widely recognized hereditary cancer syndrome worldwide. Identification of a *BRCA* variant not only informs targeted therapies, such as the use of poly ADP-ribose polymerase (PARP) inhibitors, but also allows risk-reducing interventions for unaffected carriers. As a result, oncologists, surgeons, and gynecologists are increasingly called upon to integrate genetic considerations into daily practice.

In Japan, these global trends are mirrored but also shaped by unique healthcare structures. Insurance reimbursement, facility requirements, and the strict definition of genetic counseling "notified facilities" have created a distinctive system with both strengths and weaknesses. This proceeding will review the increasing opportunities for hereditary cancer diagnosis globally, highlight the Japanese experience with *BRCA* testing, discuss challenges in referral and cascade testing, and describe the development of a system for remote genetic counseling. Our aim is to provide clinical practitioners with a pragmatic overview of where we stand, what barriers remain, and how these might be overcome.

2 Diagnosis of Hereditary Cancer

2.1 Increasing Opportunities for Hereditary Cancer Diagnosis Worldwide

The global expansion of hereditary cancer diagnosis has been driven by multiple factors:

1. Companion diagnostics in oncology: The approval of PARP inhibitors for *BRCA*-mutated ovarian, breast, pancreatic, and prostate cancers represented a paradigm shift [1, 2]. For the first time, germline *BRCA* status directly influenced systemic therapy. This linkage of treatment and genetics prompted oncologists to request *BRCA* testing for therapeutic purposes, often revealing hereditary cancer syndromes that might otherwise have gone unrecognized.

2. Comprehensive genomic profiling (CGP): With the advent of NGS, tumor genomic profiling panels frequently include germline analysis or identify pathogenic variants incidentally. Programs such as the NCI-MATCH trial in the United States have demonstrated the feasibility and impact of large-scale tumor genomic profiling in identifying actionable somatic alterations across diverse cancer types [3]. While NCI-MATCH primarily focused on somatic variants to guide treatment, similar profiling strategies are increasingly revealing germline mutations—such as *BRCA1/2*—as secondary findings when tumor and normal tissues are evaluated. In Japan, the introduction of Cancer Genomic Medicine (CGM) under the national health insurance system—especially the reimbursement of tumor profiling tests since June 2019—has significantly expanded access to tumor genetic assessment and the detection of potentially actionable variants [4].
3. Guideline-driven testing: International guidelines such as those from the National Comprehensive Cancer Network (NCCN) and the European Society for Medical Oncology (ESMO) recommend genetic testing for broad groups of patients with breast, ovarian, pancreatic, and prostate cancers [5, 6]. These guidelines include specific recommendations for risk-reduction and screening in hereditary breast–ovarian cancer syndromes. In the United States, a nationwide analysis found that among newly diagnosed breast cancer patients, approximately 56% underwent *BRCA* testing, with progressive increases over time—37% in earlier years rising to 68% by 2020 [7].
4. Public and patient awareness: Media coverage and advocacy have increased awareness of hereditary cancers. The well-publicized cases of individuals undergoing risk-reducing mastectomy or salpingo-oophorectomy after *BRCA* testing have shifted public perception, leading more patients to request testing.

Together, these factors have transformed hereditary cancer diagnosis from a niche service into a routine component of oncology.

2.2 Regional Differences and Health System Structures

Despite global progress, significant differences exist between countries or regions.

- United States: In the United States, insurance coverage for *BRCA* testing differs substantially between public and private payers. For example, a comparative study found that private payers typically covered *BRCA* testing for both affected and unaffected individuals with relevant personal or family history, whereas local Medicare carriers generally limited coverage to those with a personal diagnosis of cancer, and some state Medicaid programs did not cover testing at all [8].
- Western Europe: Access to *BRCA* testing and related preventive care in Europe is highly variable, reflecting differences in national health systems and reimbursement structures. Despite the existence of pan-European guidelines recommending genetic counseling and testing for women with suggestive personal or

family histories, implementation remains uneven. Cardoso et al. highlighted that outdated reimbursement systems and structural limitations represent major barriers to delivering guideline-concordant care for breast cancer patients across Europe [9]. In several countries, the lack of appropriate reimbursement codes for genetic testing and risk-reducing surgery limits the ability of clinicians to offer recommended interventions, thereby undermining equity of access.
- Asia: Kwong et al. conducted a multinational survey to evaluate the current status of *BRCA* testing and genetic counseling across Asia. There was substantial heterogeneity in service availability: while high-resource regions such as Japan, South Korea, Hong Kong, and Singapore reported relatively established genetic testing/genetic counseling programs, many other countries in South and Southeast Asia faced significant gaps. Major barriers included limited numbers of trained genetic counselors, uneven geographic distribution of services, and a lack of standardized national guidelines. In some settings, testing was restricted to academic centers or required out-of-pocket payment, creating inequities in access. Cultural factors such as reluctance to discuss hereditary risk within families, stigma, and low public awareness further limited uptake [10].

These variations highlight the importance of not only technology but also health policy, infrastructure, and cultural context in shaping hereditary cancer care.

2.3 The Japanese System for BRCA *Genetic Testing*

Japan has taken a distinctive approach to implementing *BRCA* testing within its universal health insurance framework. Unlike in some countries where testing can be ordered in any oncology or surgical clinic, in Japan, reimbursement is contingent upon meeting facility requirements.

BRCA testing is listed separately in the national fee schedule (item D006-18). To be reimbursed, testing must be performed at a hospital or clinic that is formally registered as a "notified facility" (*todokede shisetsu*) for genetic counseling. These facilities are required to employ board-certified clinical geneticists and to demonstrate the ability to provide structured pre-test and post-test counseling. The intent of this policy is to ensure quality, safeguard patients, and prevent misuse of genetic testing.

In practice, however, many hospitals that treat large numbers of breast or gynecologic cancer patients are not notified facilities. These hospitals are designated instead as "collaborating facilities." Collaborating facilities can perform *BRCA* testing, but they must do so in formal cooperation with a notified facility, which is responsible for providing or supervising the genetic counseling. The system was designed as a compromise: to allow widespread access to testing, while ensuring that high standards of counseling are maintained.

This dual structure is unique internationally. In the United States or Europe, genetic testing can be ordered in a wide range of settings, though best practice still recommends genetic counseling. Japan's regulatory framework is thus stricter, but it has created unintended consequences in the form of limited referrals and fragmented care.

A multicenter analysis using the JOHBOC[1] registry demonstrated that insurance eligibility criteria—such as age at breast cancer onset ≤45 years, TNBC ≤60 years, multiple primary breast cancers, or familial cancer history—captured individuals with pathogenic *BRCA* variants at substantially higher rates (21.1%) compared to those outside coverage (5.6%), indicating that insurance coverage conditions effectively identified candidates eligible for genetic testing [11].

2.4 Comparison with Other Hereditary Cancer Testing Systems in Japan

The contrast between *BRCA* testing and other hereditary cancer genes is instructive. Some single-gene tests (e.g., *RET, RB1, MEN1, NF1*) fall under the general genetic testing code D006-4, which requires ordering through notified facilities for genetic counseling. In contrast, *BRCA* testing, although introduced first as a companion diagnostic for PARP inhibitor therapy, can be ordered even by non-notified facilities. In this sense, the regulatory requirements for *BRCA* testing are in fact more permissive than for other hereditary cancer tests.

3 Referral to Genetic Counseling

3.1 Referral Patterns in Real-World Practice

Survey data in Hokkaido, an island in northern Japan, highlight the gap between policy design and real-world implementation. Among collaborating facilities that ordered *BRCA* testing (ordered mainly by breast surgeons), a substantial number of pathogenic variants (PVs) were identified. However, only about 25% of PV-positive patients were actually referred to a notified facility for formal genetic counseling (unpublished data).

The data collected between 2020 and 2021 illustrate this vividly. Out of 47 patients identified as PV-positive at collaborating hospitals, only 11 were referred to a notified facility. Referral rates varied significantly by geography. In Sapporo city, 9 of 20 positive cases were referred (45%), while outside the city, only 2 of 27 positive cases were referred (7%). The difference was statistically significant ($p = 0.004$).

[1] Japan Organization of Hereditary Breast and Ovarian Cancer.

This indicates that distance from urban centers is a major determinant of whether patients are connected to specialized genetic counseling. It also underscores the risk of inequity in hereditary cancer care under the current system.

3.2 Reasons for Non-referral

When collaborating facilities were asked why PV-positive patients were not referred to notified facilities, multiple reasons emerged:

- Patient refusal: Some patients declined further counseling, perceiving it as unnecessary or fearing additional emotional burden.
- Perceived lack of relatives: Physicians felt that counseling was of limited value when patients had no children or siblings.
- Poor medical condition: A severely ill patient was considered unable to travel to distant facilities.
- Other reasons: For example, patients were already receiving counseling at a non-partner institution, or they preferred not to transfer.

These findings reveal both system-level barriers (distance, facility distribution) and patient-level barriers (attitudes, health condition). They also highlight gaps in physician understanding: some providers underestimated the value of genetic counseling even in patients without close relatives, overlooking issues such as reproductive planning, psychological support, and broader family networks.

3.3 Implications for Clinical Care

The consequences of these referral patterns are profound. Without structured genetic counseling:

- Patients may not fully understand the implications of their *BRCA* result.
- Relatives may remain uninformed and miss opportunities for surveillance or preventive care.
- Psychological support may not be provided, leaving patients vulnerable to anxiety or misunderstanding.
- Coordination of cascade testing is hindered, limiting the public health impact of genetic diagnosis.

Genetic testing without genetic counseling is sometimes inadequate and potentially harmful. Yet, in Japan's current system, only a quarter of patients are offered genetic counseling. Bridging this gap is therefore a central challenge.

4 Cascade Genetic Counseling and Testing

4.1 International Uptake

The true impact of identifying a hereditary cancer syndrome lies not only in the care of the index patient but also in the opportunity to prevent cancer in at-risk relatives. Cascade genetic counseling and testing—the systematic offering of testing to family members of known carriers—has therefore become a cornerstone of hereditary cancer management.

Despite its importance, international evidence consistently shows that cascade testing uptake is disappointingly low. A systematic review and meta-analysis by Frey et al. found that, across HBOC families, the rate of relatives undergoing cascade testing was only about 40% [12]. Uptake was similarly low for Lynch syndrome and other hereditary cancer syndromes. This means that more than half of at-risk individuals remain unidentified and unprotected, even when a pathogenic variant is confirmed in their family.

In Japan, Kiyozumi et al. recently reported a retrospective study involving 125 HBOC probands and 425 of their first-degree relatives in Japan to identify factors promoting cascade genetic testing. The overall uptake among relatives was low: only 21.6% underwent testing, although most did so within 6 months of the proband's diagnosis [13].

4.2 Barriers to Cascade Testing

The reasons for this limited uptake are complex and multifactorial:

1. Communication challenges: Perhaps the most consistent barrier is the difficulty probands experience in communicating genetic test results to relatives. Many patients describe the result as "bad news" and feel burdened by the responsibility of disclosure [14]. Concerns include the following:
   - Fear of causing anxiety or distress.
   - Uncertainty about how to explain complex genetic information.
   - Worries about damaging family relationships.
   - Lack of contact with estranged relatives.
2. Psychological impact: Receiving a hereditary cancer diagnosis can trigger guilt, shame, or feelings of responsibility for transmitting risk to children [15, 16]. These emotions may inhibit open discussion. Some patients also internalize stigma, perceiving their genetic result as a personal flaw, which they hesitate to disclose.

3. System-level barriers: Even when patients wish to inform relatives, health system limitations can impede the process. Few countries have formal mechanisms for contacting relatives directly; most rely on probands to share information [12].
4. Financial barrier: The cost of cascade testing varies greatly depending on the healthcare system in each country. In Japan, testing of relatives is entirely self-funded, which is one of the barriers to testing. Furthermore, insurance coverage, costs, and logistics of testing may vary across jurisdictions, complicating uptake [17].
5. Cultural and social norms: In many Asian contexts, including Japan, maintaining family harmony is highly valued. Delivering distressing information may be seen as disruptive, leading some individuals to withhold results. In other cultures, patriarchal family structures or religious beliefs may affect communication patterns.

These barriers are not unique to HBOC but apply broadly across hereditary cancer syndromes. However, HBOC has been most studied due to its prevalence and the visibility of *BRCA* testing.

4.3 Japanese Context: Cultural and Structural Influences

In Japan, cascade testing faces the same challenges as elsewhere, compounded by cultural and systemic factors:

- Reluctance to share "bad news": Qualitative studies indicate that Japanese patients often struggle to disclose genetic risk to relatives, fearing they may "burden" others or disrupt family harmony. This aligns with broader cultural tendencies toward avoiding confrontation or distressing topics.
- Genetic discrimination concerns: Despite the enactment of laws and guidelines, fears about discrimination in employment or insurance remain. Patients may hesitate to share results lest the information spread beyond the family.
- Limited professional involvement: Japanese clinicians rarely contact relatives directly. The responsibility for disclosure falls entirely on the proband, which may overwhelm patients.
- Systemic restrictions: Because only notified facilities can provide counseling under reimbursement rules, relatives living far from such centers may face practical barriers to accessing care, even if they are informed.

These issues converge to limit cascade uptake, mirroring international data but with unique Japanese nuances.

4.4 Strategies to Overcome Barriers

Several strategies have been proposed to improve cascade uptake and mitigate psychosocial burden:

1. Direct contact by healthcare providers: In some countries, with patient consent, clinicians may contact relatives directly. This approach increases uptake but raises ethical and privacy debates [12].
2. Structured information tools: Written family letters, standardized information sheets, and digital resources can support patients in explaining results to relatives.
3. Psychological support integrated with counseling: Embedding mental health assessment and support within genetic services helps address guilt, anxiety, and family conflict.
4. Telemedicine approaches: The usefulness of remote genetic counseling, especially for patients living in remote areas, has already been demonstrated [18]. This method will also improve access to genetic counseling for relatives living in different regions from the patient.
5. Nationwide standardization: Standardization of cascade testing processes, adjusting legal and ethical frameworks to accommodate direct contact while respecting privacy laws, is essential.

In Japan, these strategies have only begun to be explored. A multilevel approach that combines direct contact, educational interventions, and system-level reforms to help overcome barriers to cascade testing. Among those, remote genetic counseling may offer a particularly valuable tool in overcoming geographic and cultural barriers.

5 Remote Genetic Counseling

5.1 Japan's Insurance Framework

Recognizing the challenges of geography and limited manpower, Japan has introduced reimbursement for remote collaborative genetic counseling. Under this model, counseling can be delivered via telemedicine, with a local physician physically present with the patient while a genetic specialist joins remotely. This model is referred to as Dr. to Patient with Dr. and is designed to ensure both quality and accessibility.

However, the scope of insurance coverage is restricted. Currently, reimbursed remote counseling applies only to rare diseases designated under the national scheme. HBOC, despite being one of the most common hereditary cancer syndromes, is excluded. This exclusion reflects the historical categorization of HBOC not as a rare disease but as a relatively prevalent hereditary cancer syndrome.

Ironically, this leaves the most frequently encountered hereditary condition without access to the most needed remote support system.

5.2 Development of a Self-Funded Remote Counseling System

To address this gap, we developed and implemented a remote genetic counseling system specifically for HBOC. The system connects collaborating hospitals with our hospital via a secure telemedicine platform. The counseling is provided in a Dr. to Patient with Dr. format: the patient is in the local collaborating hospital with their treating physician, while a geneticist of our hospital joins remotely.

The system was designed with several key objectives:

1. Accessibility: enable patients in rural or underserved areas to receive high-quality genetic counseling without traveling long distances.
2. Integration: ensure that genetic counseling is directly tied into ongoing oncology care by involving the local physician.
3. Education: expose local healthcare professionals to the genetic counseling process, thereby increasing their understanding and capacity.
4. Family involvement: allow geographically dispersed relatives to join sessions remotely.

Early implementation has demonstrated feasibility and patient satisfaction, though systematic evaluation is ongoing.

5.3 Advantages of the Self-Funded Model

The self-funded remote counseling system offers multiple advantages:

- Improved access: Patients who previously would not have traveled to a notified facility can now receive counseling.
- Continuity of care: The presence of the local physician ensures that genetic information is immediately contextualized within treatment plans.
- Knowledge transfer: Local clinicians observe the process and gain experience, fostering broader expertise.
- Family participation: Remote sessions allow family members in different regions to join, supporting cascade communication.

5.4 Disadvantages and Challenges

Nonetheless, there are important limitations:

- Financial burden: Because the system is not reimbursed, patients must pay the fee out-of-pocket. Although costs are modest compared to international standards, they remain a barrier.
- Technical issues: Internet connectivity, lack of non-verbal cues, and difficulty sharing documents or images can impair communication.
- Administrative complexity: Establishing contracts, billing processes, and workflows between institutions requires significant effort.
- Follow-up care: Ensuring psychological support and long-term follow-up remains challenging if local resources are limited.

These disadvantages highlight the need for policy change to extend insurance reimbursement to HBOC and other common hereditary cancers.

6 Future Perspectives

The future of hereditary cancer care in Japan will depend on addressing both systemic and cultural barriers. Several directions are evident:

1. Policy reform: Expanding insurance coverage for remote counseling to include HBOC is a critical priority. This would reduce financial inequities and align reimbursement with clinical need.
2. Network expansion: Building larger networks of collaborating hospitals will enable standardized care pathways across regions.
3. Digital innovation: Enhancing telemedicine platforms to better convey nonverbal cues, integrate educational resources, and allow secure family participation.
4. Integration with psycho-oncology: Embedding routine psychological assessment and support into genetic counseling services.
5. International collaboration: Learning from countries that have implemented direct-contact approaches or national cascade programs to improve uptake.

Ultimately, the goal is to create a seamless, equitable system in which every patient and family affected by hereditary cancer can access timely counseling, testing, and support.

7 Conclusion

The opportunities to diagnose hereditary cancer syndromes have expanded rapidly, driven by companion diagnostics, genomic profiling, and growing awareness. In Japan, *BRCA* testing has become central to oncology but is constrained by unique facility requirements that limit referral and counseling. Real-world data show that only about 25% of pathogenic variant–positive patients at collaborating hospitals are referred to notified facilities.

Internationally, cascade testing uptake remains low, around 40%, due to communication difficulties, psychological burden, and cultural barriers. In Japan, reluctance to share "bad news," concerns about discrimination, and geographic inequities further compound the problem.

Although Japan's insurance system supports remote counseling for rare diseases, HBOC is excluded. To fill this gap, we have developed a self-funded remote counseling model that connects hospitals via telemedicine in a Dr-to-Patient with Dr. format. This system offers significant advantages in access, integration, and education but also poses challenges of cost and sustainability.

The path forward will require policy reform, technological innovation, and expanded networks. By addressing both systemic and psychosocial barriers, we can move toward a future in which hereditary cancer care is accessible, equitable, and effective for all patients and families.

References

1. Robson M, Im S-A, Senkus E, Xu B, Domchek SM, et al. Olaparib for metastatic breast cancer in patients with a germline BRCA mutation. N Engl J Med. 2017;377(6):523–33.
2. Moore K, Colombo N, Scambia G, Kim B-G, Oaknin A, et al. Maintenance olaparib in patients with newly diagnosed advanced ovarian cancer. N Engl J Med. 2018;379(26):2495–505.
3. Flaherty KT, Gray RJ, Chen AP, Li S, McShane LM, et al. Molecular landscape and actionable alterations in a genomically guided cancer clinical trial: National Cancer Institute molecular analysis for therapy choice (NCI-MATCH). J Clin Oncol. 2020;38(33):3883–94.
4. Mukai Y, Ueno H. Establishment and implementation of cancer genomic medicine in Japan. Cancer Sci. 2021;112(3):970–7.
5. NCCN Clinical Practice Guidelines in Oncology: Genetic/Familial High-Risk Assessment: Breast, Ovarian, Pancreatic, and Prostate. Version 1.2026. Available from: chrome-extension://efaidnbmnnnibpcajpcglclefindmkaj/https://www.nccn.org/professionals/physician_gls/pdf/genetics_bopp.pdf/. Last accessed 01/23/2026.
6. Sessa C, Balmana J, Bober SL, Cardoso MJ, Colombo N, et al. Risk reduction and screening of cancer in hereditary breast-ovarian cancer syndromes: ESMO clinical practice guideline. Ann Oncol. 2023;34(1):33–47.
7. Centers for Disease Control and Prevention. Persistent underutilization of genetic testing for hereditary cancer. Genomics and Precision Health Blog. 2023 Jul 25. Available from: https://blogs.cdc.gov/genomics/2023/07/25/persistent-underutilization/. Last accessed 01/23/2026.
8. Wang G, Beattie MS, Ponce NA, Phillips KA. Eligibility criteria in private and public coverage policies for BRCA genetic testing and genetic counseling. Genet Med. 2011;13(12):1045–50.
9. Cardoso F, MacNeill F, Penault-Llorca F, Eniu A, Sardanelli F, et al. Why is appropriate healthcare inaccessible for many European breast cancer patients?—the EBCC 12 manifesto. Breast. 2021;55:128–35.
10. Kwong A, Tan DSP, Ryu JM, ACROSS Consortium. Current practices and challenges in genetic testing and counseling for women with breast and ovarian cancer in Asia. Asia Pac. J Clin Oncol. 2025;21(2):211–20.
11. Takahashi M, Minoura Y, Den H, Nomizu T, Ishida T, et al. Analysis of the conditions for applying BRCA genetic testing to women with breast cancer using the Japanese HBOC

consortium and the Japanese organization of hereditary breast and ovarian cancer (JOHBOC) registry project database. Breast Cancer. 2025;32(4):792–802.
12. Frey MK, Ahsan MD, Bergeron H, Lin J, Li X, et al. Cascade testing for hereditary cancer syndromes: should we move toward direct relative contact? A systematic review and meta-analysis. J Clin Oncol. 2022;40(35):4129–43.
13. Kiyozumi Y, Nishimura S, Kado N, Higashigawa S, Horiuchi Y, et al. Factors affecting the implementation of cascade testing of patients with BRCA1 or BRCA2 pathogenic germline variants in Japan. J Genet Couns. 2025;34(3):e70055.
14. Forrest LE, Delatycki MB, Skene L, Aitken M. Communicating genetic information in families — a review of guidelines and position papers. Eur J Hum Genet. 2007;15(6):612–8.
15. Ringwald J, Wochnowski C, Bosse K, Giel KE, Schaffeler N et al. Psychological distress, anxiety, and depression of cancer-affected BRCA1/2 mutation carriers: a systematic review. J Genet Counsel 2016;25(5):880–891, J Genet Couns.
16. Hamilton JG, Lobel M, Moyer A. Emotional distress following genetic testing for hereditary breast and ovarian cancer: a meta-analytic review. Health Psychol. 2009;28(4):510–8.
17. Levine R, Kahn RM, Perez L, Brewer J, Ratner S, et al. Cascade genetic testing for hereditary cancer syndromes: a review of barriers and breakthroughs. Fam Cancer. 2024;23(2):111–20.
18. Fournier DM, Bazzell AF, Dains JE. Comparing outcomes of genetic counseling options in breast and ovarian cancer: an integrative review. Oncol Nurs Forum. 2018;45(1):96–105.

Update on Evaluation of Homologous Recombination Deficiency (HRD)

Current Status and Problems of HRD Testing in Ovarian Cancer Treatment

Koji Nishino

Abstract HRD is a useful biomarker, positive in approximately 50–60% of advanced ovarian cancer. Since maintenance therapy with PARP inhibitors offers significant survival benefit, especially in HRD-positive tumors, physicians treating ovarian cancer patients must accurately and appropriately identify HRD-positive ovarian cancer.

However, HRD assays also have several limitations in identifying HRD-positive ovarian cancer, including issues with the MyChoice® GIS cutoff value, the existence of alternative evaluation methods other than MyChoice®, and problems related to tumor heterogeneity and changing HRD score over time. Furthermore, we must recognize that HRD testing is also a genetic test that can help identify HBOC.

Keywords Ovarian cancer · HRD · GIS cutoff values · Tumor heterogeneity · HBOC

1 Introduction: The Impact of PARP Inhibitors on HRD Ovarian Cancer Management

Phase 3 clinical randomized trials such as SOLO1 [1], PRIMA [2], and PAOLA-1 [3] demonstrated survival benefits with maintenance treatment with PARP inhibitors in patients with advanced ovarian cancer (stage III/IV, high-grade serous, or endometrioid subtype) especially those who have germline or somatic *BRCA1/2* variants and/or homologous recombination deficiency (HRD)-positive tumors. Approximately 50–60% of advanced ovarian cancers are HRD positive [4, 5] (Fig. 1), and since PARP inhibitors are expected to provide significant survival

K. Nishino (✉)
Department of Gynecologic Oncology, Niigata Cancer Center Hospital, Niigata, Japan

Department of Familial and Hereditary Oncology (Obstetrics and Gynecology), Niigata University Graduate School of Medical and Dental Sciences, Niigata, Japan
e-mail: knishino@med.niigata-u.ac.jp

M. Arai et al. (eds.), *Practical Guide to Hereditary Breast and Ovarian Cancer IV*, https://doi.org/10.1007/978-981-95-6580-1_16

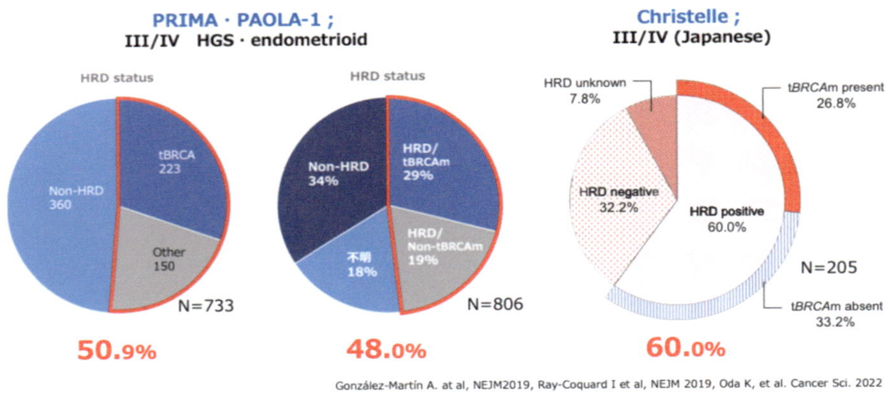

Fig. 1 Frequency of HRD in advanced ovarian cancer. The frequency of HRD was 50.9% ($N = 733$) in PRIMA and 48.0% ($N = 806$) in the PAOLA-1 trial. In the Christelle study, 60% of Japanese ovarian cancers are determined as HRD positive

benefits, it is essential to accurately and appropriately detect HRD-positive tumors within ovarian cancer patients.

2 Some Issues with HRD Testing

1. *Cutoff value of Genomic Instability Score(GIS)on Myriad MyChoice®*

   The HRD testing method approved for insurance coverage in Japan is only MyChoice® (Myriad.co.). In MyChoice®, HRD is determined when genomic DNA extracted from tumor tissue exhibits *BRCA1/2* somatic variants or when the Genomic Instability Score (GIS), evaluated by combining the three assays such as LOH (loss of heterozygosity), TAI (telomeric allelic imbalance), and LST (large-scale stage transitions), is 42pts or higher. This cutoff value of 42 was calculated by combining both ovarian and breast cancer data, however, since breast cancer has a lower GIS than ovarian cancer and the overall cutoff value is calculated to be low. Furthermore, the optimal GIS cutoff value remains unclear, as cases with *BRCA1/2* variants also exist where GIS < 42. Other studies have proposed different GIS cutoff values, such as 63 [6] or 33 [7].
2. *Diversity of evaluation methods for HRD status*

   The determination of HRD status itself involves three approaches: (1) germline/somatic variants in HR-related genes, (2) genomic instability, and (3) HR function (Fig. 2). The HRD assessment methods and GIS cutoff values adopted also vary across clinical trials.

   Sugino et al. reported the results of targeted sequencing analysis of 16 HR-related genes and 4 MMR genes in 207 ovarian cancer cases and revealed HR-related gene mutation frequencies ranging from approximately 28% to 44% among several histological subtypes [8] (Fig. 3). In this report, the HR-related

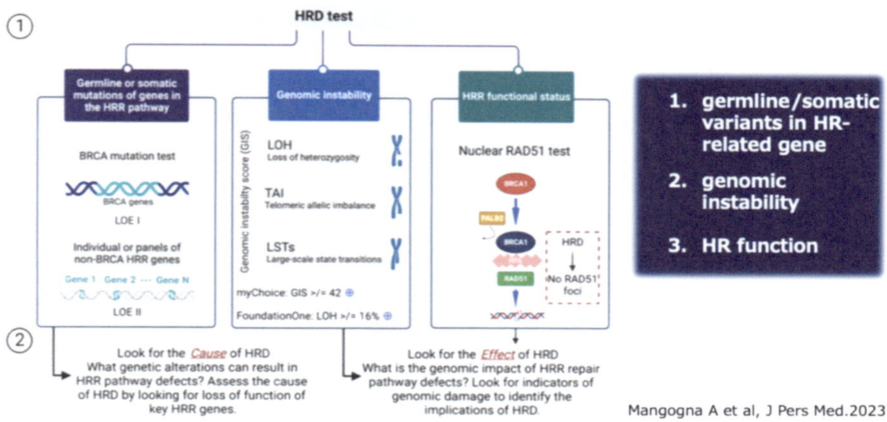

Fig. 2 The determination of HRD status. The determination of HRD status itself involves three approaches: (1) germline/somatic variants in HR-related genes, (2) genomic instability, and (3) HR function

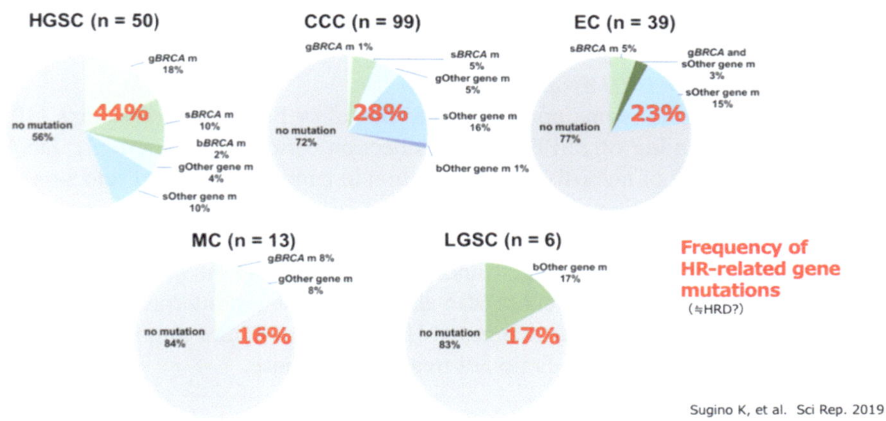

Fig. 3 Targeted sequencing analysis of 16 HR-related genes. This figure shows the frequency of HR-related gene mutation in 207 ovarian cancer cases. HR-related gene mutation frequencies range from approximately 28% to 44% among several histological subtypes

gene mutations were not associated with ovarian cancer prognosis. Factors such as the number of cases, the high proportion of early-stage cases, and the fact that these cases were from an era before PARP inhibitors were used likely contributed to this finding.

Yoshihara et al. used targeted sequencing to identify somatic mutations in 29 HR-related genes in DNA extracted from 701 ovarian cancer tissues, defining HRD positive as the presence of one or more mutations in HR-related genes [9]. In this report, FIGO stage I/II was 47.4%, III/IV was 51.6%, and histological subtypes were high-grade serous carcinoma 42.5%, clear cell carcinoma 27.0%,

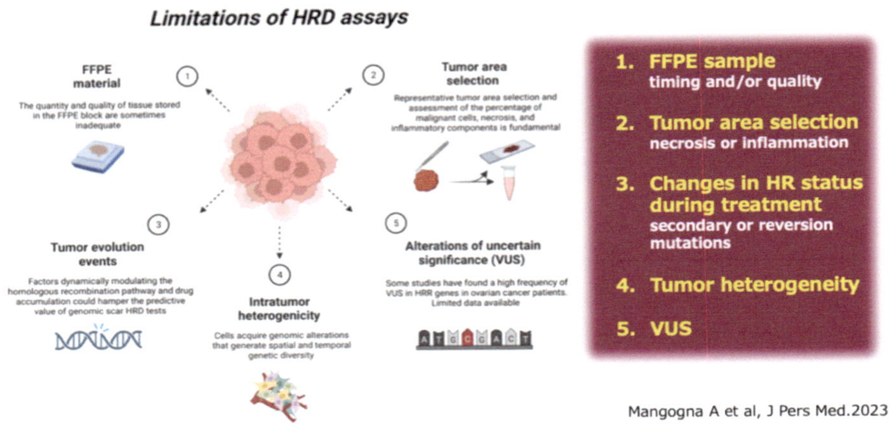

Fig. 4 Technical and biological limitations of HRD assays. There are some unavoidable technical and biological limitations in HRD testing

endometrioid carcinoma 19.3%, and mucinous carcinoma 1.7%; 42.2% of ovarian cancers were defined as HRD, and these tumors were associated with a favorable prognosis.

3. *Limitations in the HRD assay*

   HRD testing has some unavoidable technical or biological limitations [10] (Fig. 4). The timing of FFPE sample collection (primary or recurrent), DNA quality (presence of necrosis or inflammation in cancer tissue), and selection of the specimen extraction site influence the test results. HR activity during treatment may recover due to secondary or reversion mutations, which are difficult to identify by single-HRD testing. Tumor heterogeneity and the presence of VUS (variants of uncertain significance) can also complicate test interpretation. These factors may reflect temporal changes in HRD status and intra-tumoral diversity, potentially affecting the prediction of treatment response.

3 The Utility and Considerations of HRD Testing in Clinical Practice

1. *Type and sampling timing of specimen for HRD testing*

   HRD testing is possible on either surgical, biopsy, or ascites cytology specimens. The rate of "inconclusive" results is very low in surgically resected specimens from chemotherapy-naive patients. We sometimes administer neoadjuvant chemotherapy as a treatment option for advanced ovarian cancer; it is preferable to perform the HRD test on ascites or biopsy specimens before chemotherapy to obtain a reliable HRD status.

2. *Association with germline variants*

   When *BRCA1/2* somatic variants are detected within tumor tissue, 80% of these variants originate from the germline *BRCA1/2* variants, meaning they represent Hereditary Breast and Ovarian Cancer (HBOC) [11]. The relationship between *BRCA1/2* somatic and germline variants has also been demonstrated in Japanese ovarian cancer patients. Oda et al. reported that 29 of 36 t*BRCA1* variants (80.6%) and 13 of 19 t*BRCA2* variants (68.4%) in Japanese ovarian cancer patients harbored germline *BRCA1/2* variants [5]. Physicians who perform HRD testing must be aware that when t*BRCA1/2* variants are detected in some types of cancer tissue, 70–80% of these cases are HBOC who have germline *BRCA1/2* variants.

4 Conclusion

HRD status is a useful biomarker for predicting the efficacy of PARP inhibitors in the treatment of advanced ovarian cancer, contributing to improved prognosis. On the other hand, some HRD-positive ovarian cancers show resistance to PARP inhibitors and platinum, and HRD status may change during treatment, so addressing these unresolved challenges represents a critical task for the future.

References

1. Moore K, et al. Maintenance Olaparib in patients with newly diagnosed advanced ovarian cancer. N Engl J Med. 2018;379(26):2495–505. https://doi.org/10.1056/NEJMoa1810858. Epub 2018 Oct 21
2. González-Martín A, et al. Niraparib in patients with newly diagnosed advanced ovarian cancer. N Engl J Med. 2019;381(25):2391–402. https://doi.org/10.1056/NEJMoa1910962. Epub 2019 Sep 28
3. Ray-Coquard I, et al. Olaparib plus bevacizumab as first-line maintenance in ovarian cancer. N Engl J Med. 2019;381(25):2416–28. https://doi.org/10.1056/NEJMoa1911361.
4. Cancer Genome Atlas Research Network. Integrated genomic analyses of ovarian carcinoma. Nature. 2011;474(7353):609–15. https://doi.org/10.1038/nature10166.
5. Oda K, et al. Japanese nationwide observational multicenter study of tumor BRCA1/2 variant testing in advanced ovarian cancer. Cancer Sci. 2023;114(1):271–80. https://doi.org/10.1111/cas.15518. Epub 2022 Oct 18
6. Takaya H, et al. Homologous recombination deficiency status-based classification of high-grade serous ovarian carcinoma. Sci Rep. 2020;10(1):2757. https://doi.org/10.1038/s41598-020-59671-3.
7. Coleman RL, et al. Veliparib with first-line chemotherapy and as maintenance therapy in ovarian cancer. N Engl J Med. 2019;381(25):2403–15. https://doi.org/10.1056/NEJMoa1909707. Epub 2019 Sep 28
8. Sugino K, et al. Germline and somatic mutations of homologous recombination-associated genes in Japanese ovarian cancer patients. Sci Rep. 2019;9(1):17808. https://doi.org/10.1038/s41598-019-54116-y.
9. Yoshihara K, et al. Homologous recombination inquiry through ovarian malignancy investigations: JGOG3025 Study. Cancer Sci. 2023;114(6):2515–23. https://doi.org/10.1111/cas.15747. Epub 2023 Apr 10

10. Mangogna A, et al. Homologous recombination deficiency in ovarian cancer: from the biological rationale to current diagnostic approaches. J Pers Med. 2023;13(2):284. https://doi.org/10.3390/jpm13020284.
11. Mandelker D, et al. Germline-focussed analysis of tumour-only sequencing: recommendations from the ESMO precision medicine working group. Ann Oncol. 2019;30(8):1221–31. https://doi.org/10.1093/annonc/mdz136.

Timing and Cutoff Line of My Choice HRD Test

Hidekatsu Nakai, Hisamitsu Takaya, and Noriomi Matsumura

Abstract In many ovarian cancer clinical trials, the HRD score cutoff was established based on a combined analysis of breast and ovarian cancers, using The Cancer Genome Atlas (TCGA) data and two custom SNP array panels. We examined the optimal HRD score cutoff value in HGSOC using 296 cases with SNP array and exome sequencing data from HGSOC published in TCGA.

To determine the optimal timing for HRD testing, we analyzed changes in HRD status before and after chemotherapy, as well as at initial treatment and recurrence. We analyzed intra-tumoral heterogeneity, HRD scores, and copy number variations. Analysis of these matched samples revealed a significant decrease in HRD score at IDS compared with that at initial treatment. Furthermore, there was no significant change in HRD score of matching samples between initial treatment and recurrence. Our analysis revealed that the HRD test results may be influenced by chemotherapy, necessitating careful consideration of the timing of specimen.

collection for HRD testing.

Based on these results, we proposed a hypothesis regarding the clinical course of HRD tumors, and we considered the optimal treatment strategy gynecologic oncologists should pursue in the era of PARP inhibitors.

Keywords Ovarian cancer · HRD score · Primary debulking surgery · PARP inhibitor

Multiple randomized controlled trials (RCTs) have demonstrated the efficacy of PARP inhibitors. PARP inhibitors have been shown to significantly improve the prognosis of patients with high-grade serous ovarian cancer (HGSOC) [1–3]. Although the MyChoice HRD test is used as a companion diagnostic tool for PARP inhibitors, several issues remain regarding the optimal cutoff value and timing of testing.

H. Nakai (✉) · H. Takaya · N. Matsumura
Kindai University Faculty of Medicine, Osaka, Japan
e-mail: nakai@med.kindai.ac.jp; htakaya@med.kindai.ac.jp; noriomi@med.kindai.ac.jp

M. Arai et al. (eds.), *Practical Guide to Hereditary Breast and Ovarian Cancer IV*,
https://doi.org/10.1007/978-981-95-6580-1_17

In this study, we analyzed the expression of genes related to homologous recombination deficiency (HRD) in HGSOC and the effects of chemotherapy on prognosis. Based on these results, we discuss the treatment goals for gynecologic oncologists following the advent of PARP inhibitors.

1. We examined the optimal HRD score cutoff value for high-grade serous ovarian cancer (HGSOC) using publicly available data from The Cancer Genome Atlas (TCGA).

   The HRD score is evaluated based on three genomic instability factors: telomeric allelic imbalance, large-scale state transitions, and loss of heterozygosity. In ovarian cancer, many clinical trials have set the HRD score cutoff at 42 [4]. This value was established through a combined analysis of breast and ovarian cancers using TCGA data and two custom SNP panel arrays. It has also been reported that patients with a BRCA mutation exhibit high HRD scores. However, compared with other types of cancer, HGSOC has higher HRD scores. Therefore, the cutoff value of 42 derived from the combined analysis of breast and ovarian cancers may be too low [5]. Consequently, we used only the HGSOC data from TCGA to determine the optimal HRD score.

   We calculated HRD scores for 296 cases for which both the SNP array and exome sequencing data were available from TCGA. When we sorted these data in descending order of HRD score, patients with BRCA gene mutations clustered at scores of 63 or higher. We determined that 63 was the optimal cutoff point for HGSOC (Fig. 1) [6].

   Among TCGA cases, those with BRCA mutations but HRD scores below 63 retained the contralateral allele and may represent HR-proficient tumors. Data from 230,000 Foundation One case in which the association between BRCA1/2

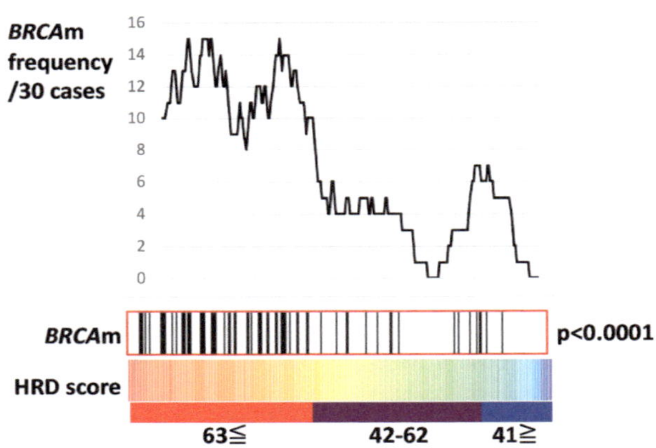

Fig. 1 Definition of HRD cases according to HRD scores. The 296 cases for which both exome sequence and SNP array data were available were sorted by HRD score. Germline *BRCA1/2* mutations and somatic *BRCA1/2* mutations are presented together as *BRCA1/2* mutations; these cases are concentrated in HRD scores ≥63. The cutoff HRD score ≥42, which is generally used, is also shown [6]

mutations and HRD status was investigated revealed that patients with BRCA mutations with loss of the contralateral allele were mostly classified as HRD tumors, whereas those with preserved contralateral alleles were less likely to be classified as such. It has therefore been reported that approximately 10% of ovarian cancers exhibit HR-proficient tumors, in which gBRCA mutations are present but the contralateral allele is preserved, thereby maintaining BRCA function. In such cases, the tumors become chemotherapy resistant despite the BRCA mutation [7].

We investigated the relationship between the HRD score and prognosis. Using the cutoff value of 63 that we proposed for the HRD score, we found that patients with a score of 63 or higher had a better prognosis than those with a score below 63, reflecting platinum sensitivity. However, when we used the previously established cutoff HRD score of 42, there was no difference in prognosis between patients with an HRD score of ≥42 and those with an HRD score of <42 [6]. Data from the prognosis analysis also suggest that an HRD score of 63 is optimal for HGSOC (Fig. 2).

2. To determine the optimal timing for HRD testing, we analyzed changes in HRD status before and after chemotherapy.

   We analyzed intra-tumoral heterogeneity, the HRD score, and copy number variation. Among patients with HGSOC treated at our institution, we examined patients whose samples were available before and after initial chemotherapy, as well as at initial treatment and recurrence. Among the HGSOC patients who underwent surgery at our institution, eight had matched samples from the initial surgery and interval debulking surgery (IDS) after chemotherapy, and six had matched samples from the initial surgery and recurrence. Analysis of these matched samples revealed a significant decrease in the HRD score at IDS compared with that at initial treatment (Fig. 3a). Furthermore, there was no significant change in the HRD score of matching samples between initial presentation and recurrence (Fig. 3b). In other words, chemotherapy caused a decrease in the HRD score, and upon recurrence, the HRD score often recovered to a value similar to that seen at initial treatment.

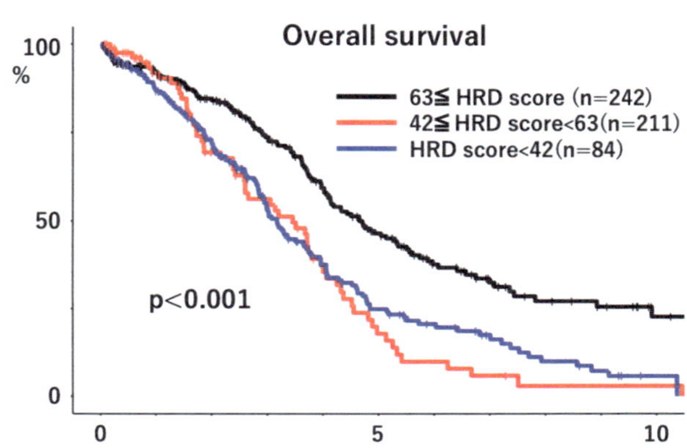

Fig. 2 Comparison of overall survival rate by HRD scores: 537 cases with known prognosis and SNP array data were divided according to HRD scores ≥63, 42–62, and ≥41 [6]

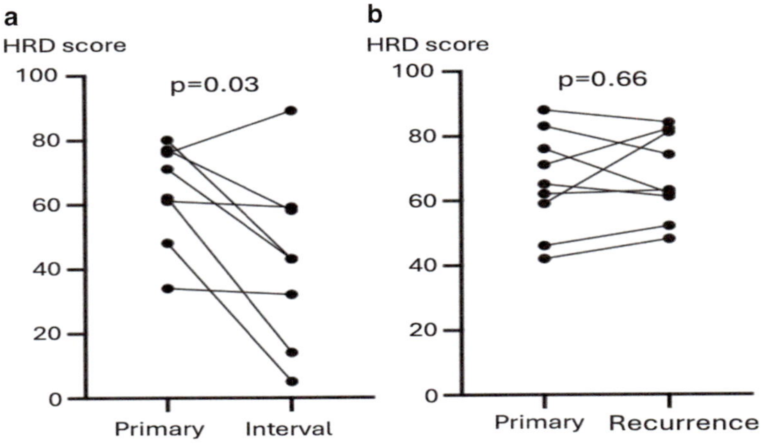

Fig. 3 (**a**) Matched samples revealed a significant decrease in HRD score at IDS compared with that at initial treatment. (**b**) No significant change in HRD score was observed between primary surgery and recurrence specimens

Table 1 Overview of the 14 HGSOC cases examined in this study

Case	Primary				Interval				Recurrence			
	BRCA1	*BRCA2*	*CCNE1*	HRD score	*BRCA1*	*BRCA2*	*CCNE1*	HRD score	*BRCA1*	*BRCA2*	*CCNE1*	HRD score
1	LOH	LOH	6	62			3	14	LOH	LOH	5	63
2	* LOH		2	76	* LOH	LOH	1	89			3	62
3	* LOH		2	71	*		2	43	LOH		2	82
4	* * LOH	LOH	5	61	* LOH	LOH	4	59	No data	No data	No data	No data
5	LOH		2	77	LOH		2	58	No data	No data	No data	No data
6			4	48			2	5	No data	No data	No data	No data
7	LOH		21	34			31	32	No data	No data	No data	No data
8	LOH	LOH	4	80			3	43	No data	No data	No data	No data
9	LOH	LOH	2	83	No data	No data	No data	No data	LOH	LOH	2	74
10	LOH	LOH	2	59	No data	No data	No data	No data	LOH	LOH	2	81
11	LOH		3	88	No data	No data	No data	No data	LOH		3	84
12	LOH		2	42	No data	No data	No data	No data			4	48
13		LOH	6	46	No data	No data	No data	No data			13	52
14	LOH	LOH	5	65	No data	No data	No data	No data			6	61

BRCA1/2 ; mutation *, LOH ■ *CCNE1* ; copy number No data ■

BRCA1/2 mutation analyses were performed for primary and initial samples.

Furthermore, we examined the HRD score, the BRCA1/2 gene mutations, and the presence or absence of BRCA1/2 loss of heterozygosity (LOH) in patients with available samples from both the initial treatment and IDS.

Specifically, in cases 1, 3, and 8, where LOH had disappeared by the time of IDS, the HRD score decreased significantly. BRCA1 gene mutations were identified in three patients, while no BRCA2 gene mutations were detected (Table 1).

All patients with BRCA gene mutations exhibited locus-specific LOH at initial treatment, but the LOH disappeared in one of three patients at the time of IDS. In case 4, two BRCA1 gene mutations were identified at the time of initial treatment; one of these mutations was lost at IDS (Table 2).

Table 2 BRCA mutations

Cases	Timing	Gene	Chr	Position	Ref.	Alt.	variant Classification	VAF (%)	LOH	HGVSG
2	Primary	*BRCA1*	17	41,244,748	G	A	Nonsense mutation	79	Yes	c.2659C > T
2	Interval	*BRCA1*	17	41,244,748	G	A	Nonsense mutation	80	Yes	c.2659C > T
3	Primary	*BRCA1*	17	41,222,965	CCAGA	C	Frameshift deletion	93	Yes	c.4822_4825del
3	Interval	*BRCA1*	17	41,222,965	CCAGA	C	Frameshift deletion	66	No	c.4822_4825del
4	Primary	*BRCA1*	17	41,246,420	A	ATT	Frameshift insertion	34	Yes	c.986_987insAA
4	Primary	*BRCA1*	17	41,267,797	CCAGA	T	Splice site mutation	32	Yes	
4	Interval	*BRCA1*	17	41,246,420	A	ATT	Frameshift insertion	65	Yes	c.986_987insAA

In case 3 with a *BRCA1* mutation, the LOH of the *BRCA1* gene was lost in the IDS specimen
Case 4 with two *BRCA1* mutations in the primary surgery specimen had one mutation in the IDS specimen

Based on these results, some tumors with high HRD scores and chemotherapy sensitivity prior to treatment subsequently exhibited reduced HRD scores and developed chemotherapy resistance. Furthermore, LOH was observed in these patients before chemotherapy but was no longer detected afterward, suggesting that this contributed to the reduced HRD scores.

Additionally, copy number alterations were lower at the time of IDS compared with those at the time of initial treatment and, upon recurrence, returned to levels similar to those at the initial treatment (Fig. 4).

Therefore, despite originating from the same patient, it was hypothesized that the tumors may have transitioned from treatment sensitive to treatment resistant between the initial treatment and the IDS stage. These findings indicate that the HRD test results may be influenced by chemotherapy, necessitating careful consideration of the timing of specimen collection for HRD testing.

3. Based on these results, we consider the optimal treatment strategy that gynecological oncologists should pursue in the era of PARP inhibitors.

   Similar reports exist regarding changes in LOH status before and after chemotherapy using samples from the same patients [8]. In this report, exome sequencing was performed before and after chemotherapy in patients with ovarian cancers with gBRCA1 mutations. Among the 11 patients in the initial treatment group, all tumors exhibited LOH for the BRCA1 wild-type allele and were chemotherapy-sensitive. However, in six of the eight patients whose tumors were resected after chemotherapy during IDS, the BRCA1 wild-type allele was retained. These findings suggest that tumor cells retaining the wild-type allele were initially present and evolved into platinum-resistant tumor cells harboring the wild-type allele during IDS after chemotherapy in gBRCA1-mutated tumors. Furthermore, it has been reported that of the six cases in which the wild-type allele was retained at the time of IDS, five subsequently recurred as chemotherapy-sensitive tumors with a LOH for the wild-type allele, which is consistent with our findings.

   To explain these results, we proposed a hypothesis regarding the clinical course of HRD tumors. First, tumor cells exhibit only minor abnormalities in the HR pathway, such as a unilaterally inherited gBRCA mutation in addition to a TP53 mutation. This state preserves homologous recombination repair function, which would classify the tumor as HR-proficient (HRP tumor). In this context, when HRD tumor cells arise—for example, due to LOH in the contralateral allele—the DNA undergoes progressive changes with each replication cycle, leading to tumor heterogeneity. Consequently, tumor cells with faster proliferation rates are selected from this heterogeneous population and expand, reaching a detectable size, resulting in the formation of primary ovarian cancer. Thus, this tumor is considered to have a high proportion of HRD tumor cells.

   When chemotherapy is administered, HRD tumor cells that are sensitive to chemotherapy are eliminated, leaving only HR-proficient, chemotherapy-resistant tumor cells. Upon recurrence, HRD tumor cells proliferate again, leading to platinum-sensitive recurrent tumors (Fig. 5).

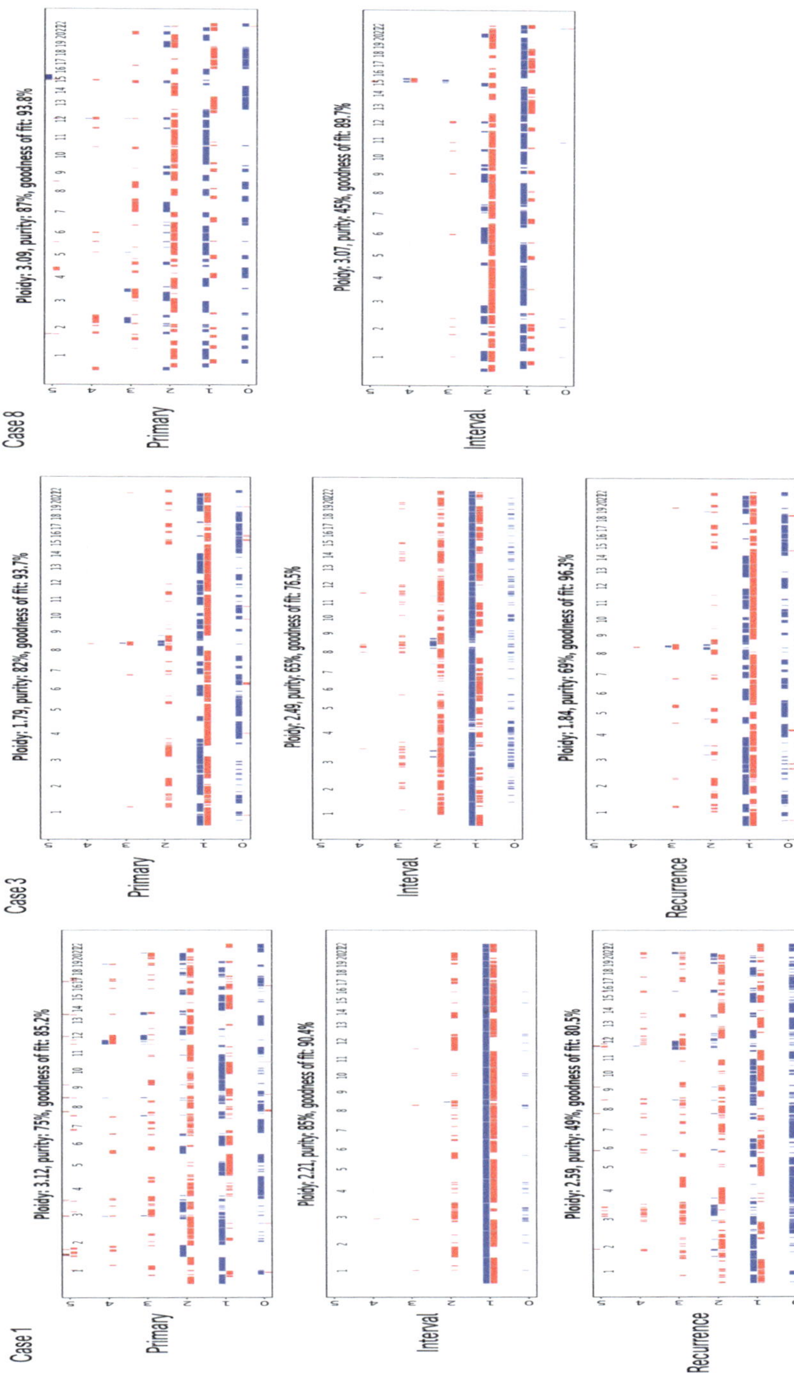

Fig. 4 Allele-specific copy number variation analysis. Representative cases are shown. IDS specimens tend to have few copy number variations

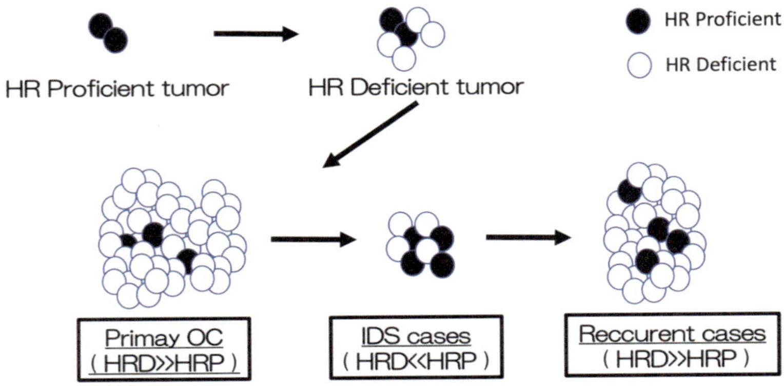

Fig. 5 We developed a model to estimate HRD status in ovarian cancer. Primary ovarian cancers are predominantly made up of HRD tumor cells. In IDS cases, the proportion of HRP tumor cells increases due to the effects of chemotherapy. At recurrence, the tumor composition shifts back to being predominantly HRD tumor cells

In other words, HRD tumors are more common in primary ovarian cancer during treatment. Chemotherapy eliminates chemotherapy-sensitive tumors, whereas IDS increases the proportion of HRP, chemotherapy-resistant tumors. At recurrence, the proportion of chemotherapy-sensitive HRD tumors may increase again.

Based on this hypothesis, we considered the clinical significance of surgery for ovarian cancer.

In accordance with our hypothesis, primary ovarian tumors constitute a high proportion of HRD tumors. If such tumors are resected macroscopically with no residual tumor, it is highly likely that only HRD tumors—i.e., chemotherapy-sensitive tumors—remain at the cellular level; this would theoretically make achieving a cure with PARP inhibitors feasible. Conversely, if surgery leaves residual tumor, the likelihood of HRP tumor persistence increases, making eradication with PARP inhibitors difficult.

However, in patients who undergo IDS after chemotherapy, the proportion of HRP tumors is high. Even if such tumors are resected macroscopically without visible residual disease, any remaining tumor cells are more likely to be HRP than PDS, making eradication with PARP inhibitors difficult.

In other words, surgery that leaves no residual tumor is considered the most effective way to minimize residual HRD tumors, particularly in PDS, which has the highest proportion of HRD tumors.

TCGA data include all PDS cases and focus on patients who did not receive molecularly targeted therapy during initial treatment. Classification by HRD status among these patients with residual tumors revealed that even the most favorable genetic-HRD group had a poor prognosis, with only approximately 30% expected to survive long term (Fig. 6a). However, when focusing only on patients

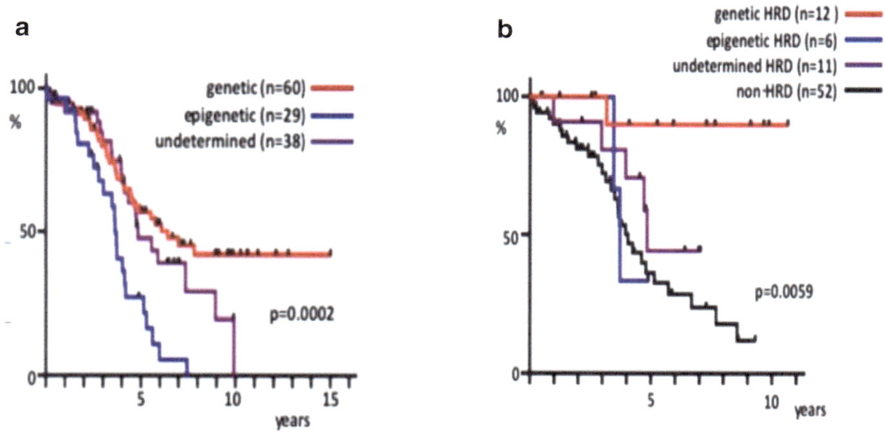

Fig. 6 Relationship among residual tumors at the time of surgery, HRD status, and prognosis. (**a**) Cases with residual tumor ≥1 mm and available SNP array data were divided into the HRD and non-HRD groups. HRD cases with exome sequencing data were further sorted by molecular mechanism into genetic HRD, epigenetic HRD, and undetermined HRD to compare the survival rate. (**b**) Similarly, cases with no macroscopic disease were classified by the HRD status for survival rate comparison [6]

with no macroscopic residual disease, genetic HRD was the only factor associated with a favorable prognosis (Fig. 6b) [6].

If the residual tumor is HRD, as per the earlier hypothesis, adding a PARP inhibitor could increase the number of HGSOC cases where a "cure" is achievable. A subanalysis of the PAOLA-1 trial reported favorable outcomes for patients with HRD, PDS, and $R = 0$ who received bevacizumab plus olaparib [9]. These findings support the hypothesis that targeting HRD tumors at the cellular level with PARP inhibitors after surgery could achieve a cure in genetic-HRD $R = 0$ cases.

These results suggest that chemotherapy in HRD tumors may reduce the number of chemotherapy-sensitive clones while increasing the proportion of chemotherapy-resistant clones. With respect to gynecological oncologists, we consider the therapeutic goal of achieving a "cure" in HGSOC to involve complete resection during initial surgery when the proportion of treatment-resistant clones is low, followed by targeting the remaining treatment-sensitive clones at the cellular level with PARP inhibitors.

Competing Interests N Matsumura has received a research grant from AstraZeneca as well as lecture fees from AstraZeneca, Takeda Pharmaceutical, Eisai, Merck Sharp & Dohme, and Chugai Pharmaceutical and is an outside director of Takara Bio. The authors have no other relevant affiliations or financial involvement with any organization or entity with a financial interest in or financial conflict with the subject matter or materials discussed in the manuscript apart from those disclosed.

References

1. Moore K, Colombo N, Scambia G, Kim BG, Oaknin A, Friedlander M, et al. Maintenance Olaparib in patients with newly diagnosed advanced ovarian cancer. N Engl J Med. 2018;379:2495–505.
2. Ray-Coquard I, Pautier P, Pignata S, Pérol D, González-Martín A, Berger R, et al. N Engl J Med. 2019;381:2416–28.
3. González-Martín A, Pothuri B, Vergote I, DePont Christensen R, Graybill W, Mirza MR, et al. Niraparib in patients with newly diagnosed advanced ovarian cancer. N Engl J Med. 2019;381:2391–402.
4. Telli ML, Timms KM, Reid J, Hennessy B, Mills GB, Jensen KC, et al. Homologous recombination deficiency (HRD) score predicts response to platinum-containing Neoadjuvant chemotherapy in patients with triple-negative breast cancer. Clin Cancer Res. 2016;22:3764–73.
5. Marquard AM, Eklund AC, Joshi T, Krzystanek M, Favero F, Wang ZC, et al. Pan-cancer analysis of genomic scar signatures associated with homologous recombination deficiency suggests novel indications for existing cancer drugs. Biomark Res. 2015;3:9.
6. Takaya H, Nakai H, Takamatsu S, Mandai M, Matsumura N. Homologous recombination deficiency status-based classification of high-grade serous ovarian carcinoma. Sci Rep. 2020;10:2757.
7. Sokol ES, Pavlick D, Khiabanian H, Frampton GM, Ross JS, Gregg JP, et al. Pan-cancer analysis of BRCA1 and BRCA2 genomic alterations and their association with genomic instability as measured by genome-wide loss of heterozygosity. JCO Precis Oncol. 2020;4:442–65.
8. Sokolenko AP, Bizin IV, Preobrazhenskaya EV, Gorodnova TV, Ivantsov AO, Iyevleva AG, et al. Molecular profiles of BRCA1-associated ovarian cancer treated by platinum-based therapy: analysis of primary, residual and relapsed tumors. Int J Cancer. 2020;146:1879–88.
9. Lorusso D, Mouret-Reynier MA, Harter P, Cropet C, Caballero C, Wolfrum-Ristau P, et al. Updated progression-free survival and final overall survival with maintenance olaparib plus bevacizumab according to clinical risk in patients with newly diagnosed advanced ovarian cancer in the phase III PAOLA-1/ENGOT-ov25 trial. Int J Gynecol Cancer. 2024;34:550–8.

A Review of Pathological Classification by Artificial Intelligence: A Challenge to HRD Diagnosis

Junzo Hamanishi, Kohei Hamada, Akihiko Ueda, and Masaki Mandai

Abstract Homologous recombination deficiency (HRD) is a crucial biomarker for guiding treatment in breast and ovarian cancers, but current molecular tests are often costly and time-consuming. This review examines three key studies that explore innovative approaches to HRD diagnosis. The potential of artificial intelligence (AI)-based deep learning shows that a model trained on standard histopathological images can predict HRD and correlate with better clinical outcomes in patients treated with platinum-based therapies. And this model identified a broader, functionally relevant HRD phenotype than traditional methods, potentially expanding the patient population eligible for treatment.

The other study highlights a major challenge: model generalizability. Their model, while effective on an internal dataset, showed a significant drop in performance on an external cohort due to technical and biological variability. This underscores the need for larger, multi-institutional datasets for robust clinical translation. Complementing these AI-based approaches, a third study presents a novel functional assay that directly measures a tumor's current HR capacity. This approach offers a valuable alternative by providing a real-time snapshot of tumor biology, which may be more reflective of chemosensitivity than historical genomic alterations.

Together, these studies suggest a synergistic future for HRD diagnosis, where AI tools serve as a rapid, accessible screening method, and functional or traditional molecular tests are used for confirmation. The goal is to develop robust, generaliz-

J. Hamanishi (✉)
Department of Obstetrics and Gynecology, National Hospital Organization Kyoto Medical Center, Kyoto, Japan

Department of Gynecology and Obstetrics, Kyoto University Graduate School of Medicine, Kyoto, Japan
e-mail: jnkhmns@kuhp.kyoto-u.ac.jp

K. Hamada · A. Ueda · M. Mandai
Department of Gynecology and Obstetrics, Kyoto University Graduate School of Medicine, Kyoto, Japan

M. Arai et al. (eds.), *Practical Guide to Hereditary Breast and Ovarian Cancer IV*,
https://doi.org/10.1007/978-981-95-6580-1_18

able AI models that can fundamentally change precision oncology and democratize access to life-saving treatments.

Keywords Ovarian cancer · Homologous recombination deficiency (HRD) · Artificial intelligence (AI) · Hematoxylin and eosin (H&E) staining · Poly (ADP-ribose) polymerase (PARP) inhibitor

1 Introduction

Homologous recombination deficiency (HRD) is a critical and well-established biomarker in oncology, particularly for patients with breast cancer and high-grade serous ovarian cancer (HGSC). Tumors that harbor HRD exhibit a profound and often exquisite sensitivity to DNA-damaging agents, including platinum-based chemotherapies and poly(ADP-ribose) polymerase (PARP) inhibitors [1–3]. This is because their compromised ability to repair DNA double-strand breaks leaves them highly dependent on alternative, often less efficient, repair pathways, which can be therapeutically targeted. Consequently, the accurate and timely identification of HRD status is paramount for guiding personalized treatment strategies and, ultimately, for improving patient survival and quality of life. Current diagnostic practices for HRD are predominantly reliant on complex and resource-intensive molecular profiling techniques. These include the detection of germline and somatic BRCA1/2 mutations, the assessment of large-scale genomic instability using genomic scar assays (e.g., Myriad's MyChoice HRD Plus), and the analysis of other relevant genetic signatures. While these methods are highly effective and provide a deep understanding of a tumor's genetic landscape, they face significant limitations [4]. They are often costly, not universally accessible in many healthcare systems, and require specialized laboratory infrastructure, which can result in diagnostic delays that may impede timely therapeutic intervention.

The burgeoning field of artificial intelligence (AI), particularly deep learning, offers a transformative and promising alternative. AI models trained on routine histopathological images, such as hematoxylin and eosin (H&E)-stained slides, have the potential to infer a tumor's molecular and functional characteristics directly from its morphological and textural patterns [5]. This innovative approach could fundamentally change the HRD diagnostic paradigm, making it faster, more cost-effective, and more broadly available across the globe. By bypassing the need for complex molecular tests, AI-based classification has the potential to democratize access to precision oncology. This review synthesizes and critically analyzes three seminal studies that explore the use of AI and novel pathological methods for HRD diagnosis, highlighting both the immense opportunities and the inherent challenges that lie within this rapidly evolving landscape [6] (Fig. 1).

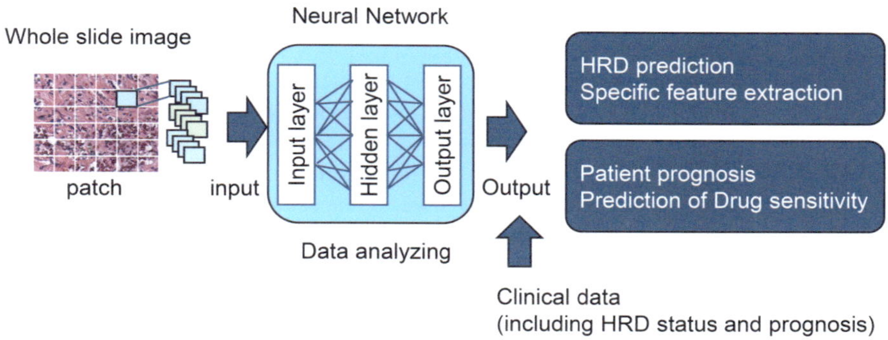

Fig. 1 The image of pathological artificial intelligence for humorous recombination deficiency in ovarian cancer by hematoxylin-eosin staining

2 Deep Learning for HRD Prediction from H&E Slides

Two recent and highly impactful studies, one by Bergstrom et al. [7] and another by Marméa et al. [8], provide compelling evidence for the potential of using deep learning on H&E-stained slides to predict HRD. They also serve as important cautionary tales regarding the challenges of clinical translation. Both research groups aimed to extract predictive features directly from the subtle morphological and textural patterns visible to AI, thereby circumventing the need for conventional molecular testing.

Bergstrom et al. developed a deep learning platform named DeepHRD, specifically designed to predict HRD from H&E-stained histopathological slides. They trained their model on a large and well-characterized dataset from The Cancer Genome Atlas (TCGA), including primary breast cancer (n = 1008) and ovarian cancer (n = 459) specimens [7]. The authors demonstrated that DeepHRD could predict HRD in a held-out breast cancer cohort from TCGA with an impressive Area Under the Curve (AUC) of 0.81. This strong performance was robustly validated in two independent external cohorts of primary breast cancer, where the model achieved an AUC of 0.76 [7]. The clinical relevance of DeepHRD was further underscored in a variety of platinum-treated clinical cohorts. In a metastatic breast cancer cohort treated with platinum therapy, samples classified as HRD by DeepHRD showed a remarkable 3.7-fold increase in median progression-free survival (PFS) (14.4 vs. 3.9 months; P = 0.0019) and a significant improvement in complete response (CR) (AUC, 0.76) [7]. Furthermore, the model's predictions correlated with better overall survival (OS) in HGSC patients treated with first-line (HR, 0.46) and neoadjuvant (HR, 0.49) platinum therapy in two separate cohorts [7]. A particularly intriguing finding from the Bergstrom study was that DeepHRD classified a substantially larger number of patients as HRD-positive (1.8- to 3.1-fold more) compared to standard molecular tests, yet these patients still experienced better clinical outcomes with platinum-based therapy [7]. This suggests that the AI model may be identifying a broader, functionally relevant HRD phenotype that is not fully captured by current genomic assays, potentially expanding the pool of patients who could benefit from these targeted treatments.

In stark contrast, the study by Marméa et al., focusing on ovarian cancer, provides a more sobering perspective. They also developed a deep learning model to predict HRD from H&E-stained whole slide images (WSIs). The model was trained on the AGO-TR1 cohort (n = 208) and externally validated on the large PAOLA-1 cohort (n = 447) [8]. While their model showed a respectable AUROC of 72% on its internal validation set, its performance dropped significantly to just 57% on the external PAOLA-1 dataset [8]. This substantial performance decay on an external cohort highlights a major, well-documented challenge in AI-based diagnostics: the issue of model generalizability. This phenomenon is often caused by technical variability, such as differences in slide scanners, tissue preparation protocols, or staining procedures, as well as biological and clinical heterogeneity between cohorts, often referred to as "dataset shift." Despite this lower predictive accuracy for HRD status itself, Marméa et al. found a clinically meaningful result. Their Kaplan-Meier analysis showed that progression-free survival in PARP inhibitor-treated PAOLA-1 patients was significantly improved in the group predicted as HRD-positive by their model [8]. This finding is crucial because it suggests that even a model with moderate predictive accuracy can still capture a true biological signal related to therapeutic benefit, indicating a potential for clinical utility even without perfect molecular correlation. The authors rightly conclude that while the development of a useful AI predictor may be possible, it will require larger cohorts and significant methodological improvements to achieve clinically viable accuracy across diverse, independent patient cohorts [8].

3 Beyond Genomics: The Importance of Functional HRD Assessment

While AI promises to infer HRD information from pathology slides, a third study by Pikkusaari et al. offers a fundamentally different and complementary approach by focusing on functional HRD assessment [9]. They developed a novel assay to directly measure the functional state of homologous recombination repair in routine formalin-fixed, paraffin-embedded (FFPE) specimens. This method quantifies RAD51, a key protein in the HR pathway, using immunostaining. By measuring RAD51 foci formation in response to DNA damage, the assay provides a real-time snapshot of the tumor's current HR capacity, which may be more reflective of its chemosensitivity than historical genomic alterations.

Pikkusaari et al. demonstrated that their functional HR (fHR) assay could significantly predict several clinical outcomes, including PFS and OS, in HGSC patients [9]. The test was effective on specimens obtained from both chemotherapy-naïve and neoadjuvant chemotherapy (NACT)-treated patients. For chemo-naïve patients, the fHR status strongly correlated with PFS ($P < 0.0001$) and OS ($P < 0.0001$), with similarly significant results for NACT-treated patients. The fHR test also successfully identified HRD in a cohort of patients who received PARP inhibitors at recurrence and subsequently experienced longer overall survival ($P = 0.0188$) [9]. This study provides a vital context for AI-based approaches. While deep learning models learn to associate morphological patterns with an HRD phenotype, the fHR assay directly measures the underlying biological function. This functional approach may be less susceptible to the variations in genomic signatures or scar scores that can be influenced by prior treatments or a tumor's specific genetic background. The authors emphasize a key limitation of existing genomic methods: they often measure "historical, not necessarily current HRD" and require a high tumor cell content, which is often not feasible for many patients [9]. A functional assay like theirs addresses these limitations and provides a compelling alternative and valuable complement to both molecular and AI-based methods.

3.1 The Integration of AI and Novel Pathology: A New Paradigm for HRD Diagnosis

These three studies collectively paint a comprehensive picture of the immense potential and the inherent challenges in using AI and novel pathological methods for HRD diagnosis. The Bergstrom et al. study provides a powerful proof-of-concept, showing that AI can predict HRD from routine H&E slides with high accuracy and clinical relevance [7]. The ability of DeepHRD to identify a larger patient population that benefits from platinum-based therapy, as compared to standard molecular tests, suggests that AI may be uncovering novel, biologically relevant phenotypes. This could lead to a significant expansion of the patient population eligible for these life-saving treatments.

However, the Marméa et al.'s study serves as a crucial reminder of the significant hurdles in translating AI models into clinical practice [7]. The substantial drop in performance on an external dataset is a persistent problem in deep learning, often caused by differences in data acquisition, cohort heterogeneity, or a phenomenon known as "dataset shift." This underscores the urgent need for larger, multi-institutional datasets and rigorous validation protocols to ensure that AI models are generalizable and reliable across diverse clinical settings.

Amidst this evolving landscape, our team is also undertaking an initiative to leverage image AI technology to evaluate tumor histopathology and homologous recombination repair deficiency status in ovarian cancer (including fallopian tube cancer and primary peritoneal cancer). We aim to clarify the dynamics of tumor immunity in cases with homologous recombination repair deficiency and construct a predictive model for treatment efficacy based on both the pathological features and immune context. This endeavor, conducted as the Japanese Gynecologic Oncology Group (JGOG3025 study), seeks to create a virtual slide data collection of tumor H&E specimens and elucidate the histopathological features associated with homologous recombination repair deficiency [10].

4 Conclusion

The integration of AI into pathology offers a truly transformative opportunity for HRD diagnosis. As demonstrated by Bergstrom et al., deep learning models can predict HRD from standard H&E slides, offering a fast, low-cost, and widely accessible alternative to complex molecular tests [7]. These models hold the potential to identify a broader patient population that benefits from targeted therapies. However, the study by Marméa et al. cautions that achieving clinically useful accuracy will require significant advancements in model generalizability and the use of larger, more diverse datasets [8]. In this context, the functional assay developed by Pikkusaari et al. provides a valuable benchmark and a complementary approach [9]. By directly measuring HR function, it offers a robust method that is less dependent on genomic signatures and potentially more reflective of a tumor's real-time response to therapy. The future of HRD diagnosis will likely involve a synergistic approach. AI-based tools could serve as a rapid, first-line screening method to identify potential HRD-positive cases, especially in resource-limited settings. For complex or equivocal cases, functional assays or traditional molecular tests could be used for confirmation. The ultimate challenge lies in developing AI models that are not only highly accurate but also robust and generalizable across different patient populations and clinical environments. As AI continues to evolve and datasets expand, it is poised to become an indispensable tool in precision oncology, fundamentally changing how we classify diseases and guide patient care.

References

1. Farmer H, McCabe N, Lord CJ, Tutt AN, Johnson DA, Richardson TB, Santarosa M, Dillon KJ, Hickson I, Knights C, Martin NM, Jackson SP, Smith GC, Ashworth A. Targeting the DNA repair defect in BRCA mutant cells as a therapeutic strategy. Nature. 2005;434(7035):917–21. https://doi.org/10.1038/nature03445. PMID: 15829967
2. Ledermann, J. • Harter, P. • Gourley, C. ... Olaparib maintenance therapy in platinum-sensitive relapsed ovarian cancer. N Engl J Med 2011; 366:1382–1392.
3. Moore KN, du Bois A. Homologous recombination deficiency testing in first-line ovarian cancer. Ann Oncol. 2022;33(3):231–3. https://doi.org/10.1016/j.annonc.2021.12.013. Epub 2022 Jan 8. PMID: 35017033
4. Mangogna A, Munari G, Pepe F, Maffii E, Giampaolino P, Ricci G, Fassan M, Malapelle U, Biffi S. Homologous recombination deficiency in ovarian cancer: from the biological rationale to current diagnostic approaches. J Pers Med. 2023;13(2):284. https://doi.org/10.3390/jpm13020284. PMID: 36836518

5. Shmatko A, Ghaffari Laleh N, Gerstung M, Kather JN. Artificial intelligence in histopathology: enhancing cancer research and clinical oncology. Nat Cancer. 2022;3(9):1026–38. https://doi.org/10.1038/s43018-022-00436-4. Epub 2022 Sep 22. PMID: 36138135
6. Guffanti F, Mengoli I, Damia G. Current HRD assays in ovarian cancer: differences, pitfalls, limitations, and novel approaches. Front Oncol. 2024;14:1405361. https://doi.org/10.3389/fonc.2024.1405361. eCollection 2024. PMID: 39220639
7. Bergstrom EN, Abbasi A, Díaz-Gay M, Galland L, Ladoire S, Lippman SM, Alexandrov LB. Deep learning artificial intelligence predicts homologous recombination deficiency and platinum response from histologic slides. J Clin Oncol. 2024;42(30):3550–60. https://doi.org/10.1200/JCO.23.02641. Epub 2024 Jul 31. PMID: 39083703
8. Marmé F, Krieghoff-Henning EI, Kiehl L, Wies C, Hauke J, Hahnen E, Harter P, Schouten PC, Brodkorb T, Kayali M, Heitz F, Zamagni C, González-Martin A, Treilleux I, Kommoss S, Prieske K, Gaiser T, Fröhling S, Ray-Coquard I, Pujade-Lauraine E, Brinker TJ. Predicting benefit from PARP inhibitors using deep learning on H&E-stained ovarian cancer slides. Eur J Cancer. 2025;216:115199. https://doi.org/10.1016/j.ejca.2024.115199. Epub 2024 Dec 26. PMID: 39742559
9. Pikkusaari S, Tumiati M, Virtanen A, Oikkonen J, Li Y, Perez-Villatoro F, Muranen T, Salko M, Huhtinen K, Kanerva A, Koskela H, Tapper J, Koivisto-Korander R, Joutsiniemi T, Haltia UM, Lassus H, Hautaniemi S, Färkkilä A, Hynninen J, Hietanen S, Carpén O, Kauppi L. Functional homologous recombination assay on FFPE specimens of advanced high-grade serous ovarian cancer predicts clinical outcomes. Clin Cancer Res. 2023;29(16):3110–23. https://doi.org/10.1158/1078-0432.CCR-22-3156. PMID: 36805632
10. Shimada M, Yoshihara K, Tanigawa T, Nomura H, Hamanishi J, Fujiwara S, Tanabe H, Kajiyama H, Mandai M, Aoki D, Enomoto T, Okamoto A. An attempt to establish real-world databases of poly(ADP-ribose) polymerase inhibitors for advanced or recurrent epithelial ovarian cancer: the Japanese Gynecologic Oncology Group. J Gynecol Oncol. 2023;34(3):e62. https://doi.org/10.3802/jgo.2023.34.e62. Epub 2023 Apr 21. PMID: 37116954

Advances in Assisted Reproductive Technology and PGT-M

Fertility Preservation in Hereditary Breast and Ovarian Cancer Syndrome (HBOC): Current Evidence and Future Perspectives

Seido Takae

Abstract Marked improvements in cancer survival among reproductive-age women have transformed fertility preservation (FP) from a niche intervention into a core pillar of survivorship care. In Japan, national policy milestones—including the Third Term of the Cancer Control Promotion Plan (2018) and the launch of a government-supported financial aid system for FP in 2021—have enabled rapid diffusion of oncofertility practices (including FP) across oncology services. The Cancer Control Promotion Plan has moved into its fourth term and is developing further (2023). Hereditary Breast and Ovarian Cancer Syndrome (HBOC), mostly caused by germline BRCA1/2 variants, represents a unique intersection of cancer genetics, reproductive endocrinology, and ethics. This scholarly review synthesizes the biological basis of female fertility, mechanisms of gonadotoxicity, and the evidence supporting established and emerging strategies for FP, with a specific focus on the care of HBOC patients. We integrate national Japanese data and programmatic advances, highlight the safety and feasibility of assisted reproductive technology (ART) in BRCA carriers, and delineate ethical and genetic counseling imperatives, including timing of risk-reducing salpingo-oophorectomy and the role of preimplantation genetic testing for monogenic disorders (PGT-M). We conclude by outlining priorities for registry-based evidence generation, equitable access, and multidisciplinary coordination that will determine the next decade of practice.

Keywords Fertility preservation · HBOC · Embryo cryopreservation · Oocyte cryopreservation · Ovarian tissue cryopreservation

S. Takae (✉)
Department of Obstetrics and Gynecology, St. Marianna University School of Medicine, Kawasaki, Japan
e-mail: s2takae@marianna-u.ac.jp

M. Arai et al. (eds.), *Practical Guide to Hereditary Breast and Ovarian Cancer IV*,
https://doi.org/10.1007/978-981-95-6580-1_19

1 Introduction

The last two decades have seen substantial gains in survival for young women with cancer due to earlier detection, optimized systemic therapy, and supportive care. However, treatments aimed at saving lives often put reproductive capacity at risk. Cytotoxic chemotherapy and pelvic radiation therapy can cause amenorrhea, premature ovarian insufficiency (POI), and long-term infertility, which can lead to serious psychosocial consequences that persist long after remission. Fertility-related psychological distress is prevalent and persistent in cancer patients and survivors [1]. Indeed, studies have shown that a very high percentage of cancer survivors experience concerns and problems related to fertility [2]. Studies consistently show that infertility treatment is always a major concern for patients of reproductive age, and timely and accurate counseling increases satisfaction and reduces decisional regret [1].

The field of oncofertility emerged to bridge oncology and reproductive medicine, ensuring that information about risks and preservation options is integrated early in cancer care. International societies—including ASCO (American Society of Clinical Oncology), ESMO (European Society for Medical Oncology), ASRM (American Society for Reproductive Medicine), and ESHRE (European Society of Human Reproduction and Embryology)—recommend that oncologists discuss gonadotoxic risk and refer eligible patients for FP before therapy begins [3]. In Japan, policy alignment has been decisive: the Third Term of the Cancer Control Promotion Plan (2018) explicitly addressed the reproductive health of adolescents and young adults with cancer, and a government-supported financial aid program for FP started in 2021, catalyzing service uptake and standardization.

HBOC patients face even more complex issues. BRCA1/2 gene mutations not only increase the lifetime risk of breast and ovarian cancer, but also, particularly in those with BRCA1 mutations, can lead to a more rapid age-related decline in ovarian reserve [4]. In addition, many will consider or undergo risk-reducing salpingo-oophorectomy (RRSO) at ages that overlap with peak reproductive years, compressing the timeline for natural conception. These realities elevate the importance of early, structured fertility counseling and, in many cases, proactive preservation. This review provides an integrated, evidence-based framework for FP in HBOC: the biology of ovarian reserve, mechanisms of treatment-related gonadotoxicity, the strengths and limitations of embryo, oocyte, ovarian tissue cryopreservation and in vitro maturation, and the safety of ART in BRCA carriers. We also summarize Japanese national data and ongoing registry efforts that will shape practice standards.

2 Biological Basis of Female Fertility

2.1 *Ovarian Reserve as the Substrate of Fertility*

Female fertility depends on a finite, nonrenewable pool of primordial follicles embedded within the ovarian cortex. Women are born with approximately 1–2 million follicles; the pool declines to ~300,000 at puberty and dwindles exponentially thereafter, with <1000 remaining near menopause [5, 6]. Because there is no conclusive human evidence to support postpartum ovarian follicle regeneration, iatrogenic loss of primordial follicles will have a permanent impact on fertility.

2.2 *Folliculogenesis and Age-Related Decline*

Folliculogenesis—from primordial recruitment to a preovulatory follicle—spans roughly six months and requires coordinated endocrine and paracrine signaling within the ovarian microenvironment [7]. Age is a factor that independently affects both the quantity and quality of eggs. In counseling, ovarian reserve markers such as antral follicle count (AFC) and anti-Müllerian hormone (AMH) are used to estimate the expected number of eggs that can be retrieved, but these do not directly measure egg quality and are merely indirect indicators. The age-related increase in aneuploidy is a critical determinant of live-birth probability [8].

3 Mechanisms of Gonadotoxicity in Cancer Therapy

3.1 *Chemotherapy*

Chemotherapeutic agents damage the ovary by inducing oocyte apoptosis, stromal fibrosis, and microvascular compromise. Alkylating agents such as cyclophosphamide and busulfan are among the most gonadotoxic due to DNA cross-linking and double-strand breaks that trigger apoptosis in primordial follicles [9]. Cumulative dose, dose intensity, and patient age modulate risk. While recovery of menses may occur in some younger women, resumption of bleeding does not guarantee preserved fecundity; primordial follicle loss can be substantial even when cycles return.

3.2 Radiotherapy

Ovarian radiosensitivity is high. Adult pelvic doses above ~6 Gy and postpubertal doses above ~10 Gy are associated with a high likelihood of permanent ovarian failure [10, 11]. Scatter from non-pelvic fields and total-body irradiation used before hematopoietic stem cell transplantation further increases risk. Ovarian transposition can reduce exposure when pelvic radiotherapy is unavoidable, but protection is incomplete if fields are extensive. Furthermore, there have been attempts to use shielding in cases of leukemia and other conditions, but from a safety standpoint, this can be considered an experimental medical treatment [12].

3.3 Pharmacologic Ovarian Suppression

Gonadotropin-releasing hormone agonists (GnRHa) administered during chemotherapy may reduce rates of treatment-induced amenorrhea in select settings, particularly hormone receptor-negative breast cancer. However, meta-analytic evidence indicates heterogeneity in effect size and uncertainty regarding improvement in live-birth outcomes [13]. On the other hand, there is also evidence that it can be used safely and increases pregnancy rates [14]. Also, large-scale domestic trials in Sweden have not provided clear evidence that GnRHa increases pregnancy rates [15]. Current consensus views GnRHa as adjunctive to—not a replacement for—cryopreservation strategies [16]. However, the most recent ASCO daily news indicates that GnRHa increases pregnancy rates, suggesting that recommendations in various guidelines may change in the future (https://dailynews.ascopubs.org/do/ovarian-protection-gnrh-agonists-during-chemotherapy-moving-evidence-routine-practice).

3.4 Risk Frameworks

ASCO and ESMO categorize gonadotoxic regimens as high, intermediate, or low risk and recommend early referral for patients in the high and many in the intermediate risk categories [3]. For breast cancer, common anthracycline- and taxane-based regimens carry intermediate risk; addition of alkylators increases risk further. Individualized risk estimates should consider age, baseline ovarian reserve, and planned radiation fields. Table 1 shows the risk classification of breast cancer treatment and fertility as presented by ASCO.

Table 1 Impact of breast cancer treatments on fertility (based on ASCO 2013 fertility preservation guideline supplement data)

Risk category	Treatment regimen/agents	Typical patient profile	ASCO 2013 notes
High risk	High-dose alkylating agent combinations (e.g., cyclophosphamide >7.5 g/m^2 in young women) or chemotherapy combined with pelvic or total body irradiation.	Patients >40 years or receiving combined chemo-radiotherapy.	Highest risk of gonadal failure and amenorrhea (>70% incidence). Fertility preservation must be discussed prior to treatment.
Intermediate risk	Standard-dose cyclophosphamide-based regimens such as AC × 4 followed by taxane (AC → T, AC → paclitaxel or docetaxel).	Women under 40 years with early-stage or locally advanced breast cancer.	Lower but significant risk of treatment-induced amenorrhea (~30–70%). Ovarian protection or fertility preservation should be considered.
Low risk	CMF, CEF, or CAF regimens (cyclophosphamide-containing protocols at standard doses).	Women <30 years with adjuvant therapy for breast cancer.	Unlikely to cause immediate amenorrhea (<30%) but may lead to earlier menopause. Fertility counseling recommended.
Very low/no risk	Non-alkylating multi-agent therapies (e.g., vincristine-based combinations without gonadotoxic drugs).	Younger patients receiving supportive or low-intensity regimens.	Negligible effect on menstrual function; fertility usually preserved.
Unknown risk	Targeted and biological agents: Trastuzumab, bevacizumab, cetuximab, imatinib, erlotinib.	HER2-positive or metastatic breast cancer patients receiving targeted therapy.	Insufficient data regarding reproductive toxicity. Fertility preservation should still be discussed prior to initiation.

Source: American Society of Clinical Oncology (ASCO) Clinical Practice Guideline Update (2013). Data Supplement #6: "Risk of Amenorrhea in Women Treated with Modern Chemotherapy and Radiotherapy." LIVESTRONG Foundation—Fertile Hope Program (Updated 2013)
This summary table is derived from the American Society of Clinical Oncology (ASCO) Clinical Practice Guideline Update (2013), Data Supplement #6: "Risk of Amenorrhea in Women Treated with Modern Chemotherapy and Radiotherapy." The table focuses specifically on breast cancer treatments and their associated risk of treatment-induced amenorrhea

4 Fertility Preservation Strategies

4.1 Embryo Cryopreservation

Embryo cryopreservation (EC) is the most established approach, offering high pregnancy rates per transfer when viable embryos are banked pre-treatment. Controlled ovarian stimulation (COS) is typically performed with antagonist protocols; in estrogen-sensitive cancers, co-administration of aromatase inhibitors such as letrozole keeps estradiol levels lower while preserving oocyte yield [17]. Fertilization can proceed via conventional insemination or ICSI, followed by blastocyst culture and vitrification. Although it is age-dependent, similar to infertility treatment, pregnancy rates per embryo transfer (ET) around 30% have been reported, with substantial cumulative live-birth rates across multiple transfers. A nationwide survey in Japan reported over 200 live births resulting from the transfer of embryos obtained through fertility preservation, with breast cancer patients accounting for the largest proportion. In breast cancer patients, the median age at egg retrieval was 37 years, and the pregnancy rate per ET was 28%, with a live birth rate of 22.5%. Notably, the live birth rate per patient was 54.9%, meaning that more than half of the patients who underwent ET successfully had a child, which is a very promising result [18].

4.2 *Oocyte Cryopreservation*

Oocyte cryopreservation (OC) has transformed outcomes: post-thaw survival rates commonly exceed 90%, with fertilization and blastocyst development approaching those of fresh oocytes. Oocyte cryopreservation enables unmarried women, or those who prefer autonomy over sperm choice, to preserve options. When sufficient mature oocytes are banked (often 8–15 or more, age-dependent), cumulative live-birth rates can approximate those of EC. Random-start protocols and, when indicated, dual stimulation within a single cycle support time-sensitive oncology workflow. A nationwide survey in Japan revealed that over 1200 OC procedures were performed in the 5 years from 2016 to the end of 2020. Although the number of ET cycles was not large at 60 cycles, the pregnancy rate was 26.8%, and the live birth rate was 17.5% (average age at the time of oocyte cryopreservation: 34.8 years). Of the patients who underwent ET after OC, 77% were breast cancer patients, with a pregnancy rate of 31.0% and a live birth rate of 21.4% per ET [19].

4.3 *Ovarian Tissue Cryopreservation*

Ovarian tissue cryopreservation (OTC) is uniquely suited to prepubertal girls and to patients who must start therapy immediately. In breast cancer patients, this is applicable to those who do not have sufficient time before the start of treatment to undergo fertility preservation procedures. Laparoscopic retrieval of cortical strips is followed by cryostorage and later autotransplantation, which can restore both endocrine function and fertility. International experience now includes more than 200 live births; restoration of menses is common, and pregnancies can occur spontaneously or via IVF [20]. In Japan, OTC is expanding but remains categorized as investigational in many centers; careful patient selection and oncologic oversight are essential. However, the latest ASCO guidelines (2025 edition) have positioned it as a clearly established medical technology in the United States [16], so its status in Japan may also change similarly in the near future. Currently, 600 cases of OTC have been performed in Japan (data provided by Professor Takai), but the number of ovarian tissue transplantations is still small [19]. Although the authors' institution has already had several live birth cases, most of them are in breast cancer patients (unpublished data).

4.4 *Counseling and Decision Support*

Counseling should explicitly address timelines, expected yields, per-cycle and cumulative probabilities, and cancer-specific safety considerations. Furthermore, the physicians and medical staff responsible for family planning need to ensure that the treatment of the tumor remains the top priority, while also guiding the patient to make choices they will not regret. Therefore, the role of the navigator is crucial. Multidisciplinary case conferences reduce delays and ensure alignment of oncologic and reproductive priorities [21].

5 Fertility Preservation in HBOC Patients

5.1 *Ovarian Reserve and BRCA Biology*

BRCA1 has a central role in homologous recombination repair. Several cohorts report lower AMH levels and earlier menopause in BRCA1 carriers relative to non-carriers, consistent with increased vulnerability of oocytes to DNA damage [22]. Evidence for BRCA2 is more mixed. These data support a lower threshold for early fertility counseling in carriers, even before any cancer diagnosis.

5.2 *Safety and Outcomes of ART in BRCA Carriers*

Concerns that ovarian stimulation might increase the incidence of ovarian or breast cancer in carriers have not been substantiated by contemporary evidence. Systematic reviews suggest no significant association between ART exposure and ovarian cancer in carriers, and pregnancy after breast cancer does not appear to worsen recurrence risk when patients are carefully selected and monitored. Limited evidence does not show an increased risk of chemotherapy-induced ovarian failure in BRCA carriers (no conclusion has been reached), but it is recommended that all women diagnosed at reproductive age should consult with their doctor about fertility preservation. Among the options, embryo and egg freezing are presented as safe methods [23]. In clinical studies, fertilization rates, blastocyst formation rates, and live birth rates are generally similar between carriers and non-carriers, but some carriers may require higher doses of gonadotropins due to reduced ovarian reserve [24, 25]. To reiterate, the views regarding ovarian reserve in BRCA carriers are controversial, and further research is needed [26, 27]. While current evidence suggests that pregnancy is safe for BRCA carriers, it would still be advisable for them to become pregnant and give birth at a younger age [23, 28, 29]. Furthermore, short-term follow-up studies (5 years) have also reported that there is no worsening of disease-free survival in BRCA carriers who undergo ART after breast cancer treatment [30]. There have also been reports regarding the safety of becoming pregnant again after being diagnosed with breast cancer during pregnancy in young women who carry the BRCA gene mutation. However, further long-term studies are needed to interpret these findings [31]. Furthermore, regarding the prognosis of BRCA carriers who become pregnant after breast cancer treatment, results from a multi-center collaborative study have shown that it does not worsen the disease-free survival period of breast cancer patients [32].

5.3 PGT-M Considerations

PGT-M allows selection of embryos that do not carry the familial BRCA variant, reducing transmission to offspring. From a medical perspective, PGT-M can be considered an effective option for patients who test positive for the BRCA gene mutation to build a family while avoiding the transmission of the genetic mutation [33]. Clinical feasibility is well established; ethical deliberation should address the nature of adult-onset cancer susceptibility, potential psychological impact, and family views. In practice, PGT-M can be empowering for some families, while others may decline based on personal values. Programs should ensure pre- and post-test genetic counseling with clear discussion of limitations, including residual cancer risk from non-BRCA pathways. Not all patients or couples necessarily undergo PGT-M. Depending on factors such as age and the resulting decrease in the number of viable embryos, there may be cases where embryo transfer is still an option even if the PGT-M results show a positive BRCA mutation [34]. We emphasize the need for genetic counseling and multidisciplinary support when considering these various options. Currently, it is difficult to perform PGT-M on embryos from BRCA carriers in Japan. It is desirable that this issue be discussed in depth not only by doctors, healthcare professionals, and patients, but also by society. Furthermore, although like the implementation of ART, the COS procedure performed to carry out PGT-M has also been reported to be safe [35].

5.4 *Ovarian Tissue Cryopreservation in Carriers*

Data on the oncologic safety of ovarian tissue autotransplantation in BRCA carriers are limited. No causal signal has emerged; nonetheless, thoughtful case selection is warranted, particularly in patients with prior ovarian or tubal neoplasia [23, 36]. Where concerns about tissue reimplantation exist, alternatives such as embryo/oocyte cryopreservation may be preferred. Research into artificial ovary constructs may eventually provide safer grafts devoid of malignant contamination risk.

6 Ethical and Genetic Considerations

6.1 *Autonomy, Beneficence, and Nonmaleficence*

FP decisions in hereditary cancer exist at the intersection of patient autonomy, clinical beneficence, and nonmaleficence. Clinicians must present risks and benefits in a balanced, comprehensible manner, including chances of success and potential delays to cancer treatment. Structured consent processes reduce decisional conflict and improve alignment with patient values.

6.2 *Genetic Counseling Across the Care Continuum*

Genetic counseling is indispensable before genetic testing, when communicating results, during FP planning, and when considering PGT-M. Counseling should clarify penetrance, variable expressivity, residual risk after RRSO, and implications for screening. For relatives, cascade testing raises additional ethical questions about privacy and responsibility.

6.3 *Equity and Access*

Financial barriers, geographic inequities, and variations in provider awareness historically limited access to oncofertility. Japan's public financial aid program significantly improves equity, but ongoing monitoring is essential to ensure that rural and socioeconomically disadvantaged populations benefit.

6.4 *Psychosocial Support*

Cancer and infertility each carry substantial psychological burden; their co-occurrence compounds distress. Integrating mental health professionals and peer support can mitigate anxiety and depression and support coping throughout treatment and family building.

7 National Evidence and Programmatic Advances in Japan

As mentioned earlier, a nationwide survey across 150 institutions between 2016 and 2020 (response rate 76%) reported 1420 EC cycles, 1273 OC, and 198 OTC cases. These FP have shown consistent reproductive outcomes. Although follow-up is still maturing, these outcomes demonstrate meaningful real-world effectiveness [18, 19]. Currently, the Japan Oncofertility Registry (JOFR) has been established, which is useful for accumulating long-term and large-scale data related to FP. JOFR provides a platform for standardized prospective data collection among participating facilities. The registry's endpoints are designed to allow for evaluation not only of clinical pregnancy rates per cycle, but also cumulative live birth rates per patient, time to ovarian function recovery, obstetric and neonatal outcomes, and long-term oncological safety [37]. In the future, it is expected that linking with genetic counseling data will enable stratified analysis of individuals carrying BRCA gene mutations and patients with other hereditary syndromes.

8 Future Directions

8.1 *Scientific Innovation*

Emerging technologies—artificial ovary scaffolds [38], in vitro folliculogenesis [39], and stem cell-derived gametes [40]—may ultimately decouple fertility from ovarian function. For HBOC, research into BRCA-related oocyte biology could yield targeted protective strategies against DNA damage. Until such advances reach clinical viability, optimizing current cryopreservation methods remains the most impactful path.

8.2 *Data, Implementation, and Learning Health Systems*

A learning-health-system approach uses routine data to drive iterative improvement. JOFR, aligned with international registries, can fuel benchmarking and meta-analysis. Transparent reporting of outcomes and complications will improve patient counseling and strengthen trust.

8.3 *Training and Culture*

Knowledge regarding oncofertility is increasingly being incorporated into oncology and gynecology training. Acquiring concise and standardized knowledge facilitates discussions about fertility and reduces missed opportunities while ensuring safety. Therefore, it is recommended to establish and actively utilize educational tools such as those mentioned above [21]. Furthermore, it is desirable to enhance training in genetics to keep pace with technological advancements and to foster a culture throughout society that allows for discussions on these topics. However, it goes without saying that these efforts must never be discriminatory.

9 Conclusion

In the care of young women with cancer, FP has evolved from an experimental stage to an essential component. In cases of HBOC, where the timeline for cancer risk and reproductive concerns often overlap, proactive counseling and timely FP can protect reproductive autonomy without compromising oncological outcomes. The safety and efficacy of EC and OC in BRCA gene mutation carriers are supported by evidence (although further long-term studies are needed). Although there is currently no positive recommendation for HBOC, OTC also expands options when time is limited or stimulation is contraindicated. The establishment of JOFR, along with government support and the efforts of academic organizations, provides a foundation for generating evidence that will serve as a standard for high-quality medical practice. Equitable access, multidisciplinary collaboration, and continued investment in patient-centered evaluation metrics will ensure that the possibility of having a family is integrated into the survivorship of those who desire it.

References

1. Logan S, Perz J, Ussher JM, Peate M, Anazodo A. Systematic review of fertility-related psychological distress in cancer patients: informing on an improved model of care. Psycho-Oncology. 2019;28(1):22–30.

2. Furui T, Takai Y, Kimura F, Kitajima M, Nakatsuka M, Morishige KI, et al. Problems of reproductive function in survivors of childhood- and adolescent and young adult-onset cancer revealed in a part of a national survey of Japan. Reprod Med Biol. 2019;18(1):105–10.
3. Loren AW, Mangu PB, Beck LN, Brennan L, Magdalinski AJ, Partridge AH, et al. Fertility preservation for patients with cancer: American Society of Clinical Oncology clinical practice guideline update. J Clin Oncol. 2013;31(19):2500–10.
4. Finch A, Valentini A, Greenblatt E, Lynch HT, Ghadirian P, Armel S, et al. Frequency of premature menopause in women who carry a BRCA1 or BRCA2 mutation. Fertil Steril. 2013;99(6):1724–8.
5. Broekmans FJ, Kwee J, Hendriks DJ, Mol BW, Lambalk CB. A systematic review of tests predicting ovarian reserve and IVF outcome. Hum Reprod Update. 2006;12(6):685–718.
6. Faddy MJ, Gosden RG. A model conforming the decline in follicle numbers to the age of menopause in women. Hum Reprod. 1996;11(7):1484–6.
7. Leung PCK, Adashi EY. The ovary. 2nd ed. Amsterdam/Boston: Elsevier; 2004. xviii, 664 p
8. te Velde ER, Pearson PL. The variability of female reproductive ageing. Hum Reprod Update. 2002;8(2):141–54.
9. Sonmezer M, Oktay K. Fertility preservation in female patients. Hum Reprod Update. 2004;10(3):251–66.
10. Meirow D, Nugent D. The effects of radiotherapy and chemotherapy on female reproduction. Hum Reprod Update. 2001;7(6):535–43.
11. Wallace WH, Thomson AB, Kelsey TW. The radiosensitivity of the human oocyte. Hum Reprod. 2003;18(1):117–21.
12. Ashizawa M, Akahoshi Y, Nakano H, Kawamura S, Takeshita J, Yoshino N, et al. Updated clinical outcomes of hematopoietic stem cell transplantation using Myeloablative total body irradiation with ovarian shielding to preserve fertility. Biol Blood Marrow Transplant. 2019;25(12):2461–7.
13. Lambertini M, Falcone T, Unger JM, Phillips KA, Del Mastro L, Moore HC. Debated role of ovarian protection with gonadotropin-releasing hormone agonists during chemotherapy for preservation of ovarian function and fertility in women with cancer. J Clin Oncol. 2017;35(7):804–5.
14. Lambertini M, Boni L, Michelotti A, Magnolfi E, Cogoni AA, Mosconi AM, et al. Long-term outcomes with pharmacological ovarian suppression during chemotherapy in premenopausal early breast cancer patients. J Natl Cancer Inst. 2022;114(3):400–8.
15. Rodriguez-Wallberg KA, Kieler H, Foukakis T, Li J, Gissler M, Oberg AS, et al. Gonadotropin releasing hormone agonist (GnRHa) during chemotherapy and post-cancer childbirths – a Nationwide population-based cohort study of 24,922 women diagnosed with cancer in Sweden. EClinicalMedicine. 2024;67:102335.
16. Su HI, Lacchetti C, Letourneau J, Partridge AH, Qamar R, Quinn GP, et al. Fertility preservation in people with cancer: ASCO guideline update. J Clin Oncol. 2025;43(12):1488–515.
17. Oktay K, Buyuk E, Libertella N, Akar M, Rosenwaks Z. Fertility preservation in breast cancer patients: a prospective controlled comparison of ovarian stimulation with tamoxifen and letrozole for embryo cryopreservation. J Clin Oncol. 2005;23(19):4347–53.
18. Takae S, Harada M, Nakamura K, Furuyama S, Ono M, Osuga Y, et al. Reproductive outcomes of embryo cryopreservation and transfer at the start-up phase of fertility preservation in Japan. Reprod Med Biol. 2024;23(1):e12581.
19. Takae S, Harada M, Nakamura K, Furuyama S, Ono M, Osuga Y, et al. Survey on the implementation status and reproductive outcomes of oocyte and ovarian tissue cryopreservation in Japan: historical comparison with nationwide surveys. J Obstet Gynaecol Res. 2024;50(4):709–18.
20. Dolmans MM, Falcone T, Patrizio P. Importance of patient selection to analyze in vitro fertilization outcome with transplanted cryopreserved ovarian tissue. Fertil Steril. 2020;114(2):279–80.
21. Ono M, Harada M, Horie A, Dai Y, Horiguchi I, Kikuchi E, et al. Effect of a web-based fertility preservation training program for medical professionals in Japan. Int J Clin Oncol. 2023;28(9):1112–20.

22. Corrado G, Marchetti C, Trozzi R, Scambia G, Fagotti A. Fertility preservation in patients with BRCA mutations or Lynch syndrome. Int J Gynecolog Cancer. 2021;31(3):332–8.
23. Buonomo B, Massarotti C, Dellino M, Anserini P, Ferrari A, Campanella M, et al. Reproductive issues in carriers of germline pathogenic variants in the BRCA1/2 genes: an expert meeting. BMC Med. 2021;19(1):205.
24. Gasparri ML, Di Micco R, Zuber V, Taghavi K, Bianchini G, Bellaminutti S, et al. Ovarian reserve of women with and without BRCA pathogenic variants: a systematic review and meta-analysis. Breast. 2021;60:155–62.
25. Turan V, Lambertini M, Lee DY, Wang E, Clatot F, Karlan BY, et al. Association of Germline BRCA pathogenic variants with diminished ovarian reserve: a meta-analysis of individual patient-level data. J Clin Oncol. 2021;39(18):2016–24.
26. Arab S, Tulandi T, Buckett W. Hereditary breast cancer and fertility preservation outcomes. J Assist Reprod Genet. 2022;39(5):1163–8.
27. Kim SW, Kim TH, Han JY, Kim SK, Lee JR, Jee UC, et al. Impact of BRCA mutations and hormone receptor status on reproductive potential in breast cancer patients undergoing fertility preservation. Gynecolog Endocrinol. 2022;38(3):227–30.
28. Maksimenko J, Irmejs A, Gardovskis J. Pregnancy after breast cancer in BRCA1/2 mutation carriers. Hered Cancer Clin Pract. 2022;20(1):3.
29. Liu X, Yue J, Pervaiz R, Zhang H, Wang L. Association between fertility treatments and breast cancer risk in women with a family history or BRCA mutations: a systematic review and meta-analysis. Front Endocrinol. 2022;13:986477.
30. Magaton IM, Blondeaux E, Hamy AS, Linn S, Bernstein-Molho R, Peccatori FA, et al. Assisted reproductive technology in young BRCA carriers with a pregnancy after breast cancer: an international cohort study. Eur J Cancer. 2025;222:115434.
31. Perachino M, Blondeaux E, Delucchi V, Bernstein Molho R, Frank S, Paluch-Shimon S, et al. Safety of having a subsequent pregnancy after prior diagnosis of breast cancer during pregnancy in young BRCA carriers. ESMO Open. 2025;10(8):105513.
32. Lambertini M, Blondeaux E, Agostinetto E, Hamy AS, Kim HJ, Di Meglio A, et al. Pregnancy after breast cancer in young BRCA carriers: an international hospital-based cohort study. JAMA. 2024;331(1):49–59.
33. Barrett F, Shaw J, Besser AG, Grifo JA, Blakemore JK. Preimplantation genetic testing for monogenic disorders: clinical experience with BRCA1 and BRCA2 from 2010-2021. J Assist Reprod Genet. 2023;40(11):2705–13.
34. Nahshon C, Lavie O, Oron G. Attitude of BRCA1/2 mutation carriers towards fertility preservation, family planning and preimplantation genetic testing for primary prevention of breast and ovarian cancer in the next generation. J Assist Reprod Genet. 2023;40(12):2835–42.
35. Wang D, Song X, Zhu X, Yan L, Zhi X, Yan J, et al. Outcomes and the effect of PGT-M in women with hormone-related hereditary tumor syndrome. Front Oncol. 2024;14:1378019.
36. Preservation EGGoFF, Anderson RA, Amant F, Braat D, D'Angelo A, Chuva de Sousa Lopes SM, et al. ESHRE guideline: female fertility preservation. Hum Reprod Open. 2020;2020(4):hoaa052.
37. Shigematsu K, Shimizu C, Furui T, Kataoka S, Kawai K, Kishida T, et al. Current status and issues of the Japan Oncofertility registry. J Adolesc Young Adult Oncol. 2022;12(4):584–91.
38. Laronda MM. Engineering a bioprosthetic ovary for fertility and hormone restoration. Theriogenology. 2020;150:8.
39. Telfer EE, Andersen CY. In vitro growth and maturation of primordial follicles and immature oocytes. Fertil Steril. 2021;115(5):1116–25.
40. Shafiei G, Talaei SA, Enderami SE, Mahabady MK, Mahabadi JA. Pluripotent stem cell-derived gametes: a gap for infertility treatment and reproductive medicine in the future. Tissue Cell. 2025;95:102904.

Progress of Discussion on Indications for PGT-M in Japan

Aiko Sasaki

Abstract Preimplantation genetic testing for monogenic disorders (PGT-M) is a rapidly evolving field that intersects with reproductive medicine, ethics, and genetic counseling. In Japan, the criteria for approving PGT-M cases have been particularly restrictive, focusing on the concept of "severe" hereditary diseases. This chapter reviews the historical background, current status, and ongoing debates surrounding the definition and scope of indications for PGT-M in Japan, with particular attention to hereditary breast and ovarian cancer (HBOC). The discussion also reflects on the societal, clinical, and policy-related factors shaping the interpretation of severity and the future direction of PGT-M eligibility.

Keywords Preimplantation genetic testing for monogenic disorders (PGT-M) · Japan Society of Obstetrics and Gynecology (JSOG) · Hereditary breast and ovarian cancer (HBOC) · *BRCA1/2* · Ethics · Severity · Reproductive autonomy

1 Introduction

Preimplantation genetic testing (PGT) encompasses a set of reproductive technologies that enable the genetic profiling of embryos prior to implantation. Among them, PGT-M is used to detect single-gene disorders in embryos created via in vitro fertilization (IVF). While widely used globally, the implementation and regulation of PGT-M differ substantially across countries. In Japan, the procedure requires approval by the relevant committee of the Japan Society of Obstetrics and Gynecology (JSOG), and the approval process has traditionally hinged on strict criteria, with a heavy emphasis on the concept of "seriousness" or "severity" of the condition.

A. Sasaki (✉)
Center for Maternal-Fetal, Neonatal and Reproductive Medicine/Center for Medical Genetics, National Center for Child Health and Development, Setagaya, Tokyo, Japan
e-mail: sasaki-a@ncchd.go.jp

M. Arai et al. (eds.), *Practical Guide to Hereditary Breast and Ovarian Cancer IV*, https://doi.org/10.1007/978-981-95-6580-1_20

This chapter aims to outline the Japanese experience in the development of PGT-M indications, focusing on ethical, clinical, and social dimensions, and to explore how the discussions have evolved over time, particularly in relation to adult-onset conditions such as HBOC.

2 Historical Overview of PGT-M in Japan

Following the publication of the "Statement on Preimplantation Diagnosis" in 1998 [1], JSOG approved approximately 120 PGT-M cases from 1999 to 2015, primarily for autosomal recessive or X-linked recessive disorders with early-onset and severe manifestations, such as Duchenne muscular dystrophy and Tay-Sachs disease [2]. At the time, the definition of "severe" hereditary disease was not formally stated in the guidelines. A turning point came in 2022, when JSOG revised its statement, formalizing the definition of severity: as a general principle, conditions in which symptoms manifest before adulthood, significantly impair daily life or pose a threat to survival, and for which there is currently no effective treatment to prevent these outcomes, or where highly intensive and invasive treatments are required [3]. This change was based on cumulative discussions in the Clinical Ethics Review Committee in JSOG since 1998, triggered in part by a 2018 application for PGT-M from a couple affected by retinoblastoma.

3 Defining "Severity" and Its Implications

The formal definition adopted in 2022 reflects a long-standing consensus: that eligible conditions must be those that manifest in childhood or adolescence, cause substantial disability or threaten survival, and lack curative or noninvasive treatments. This framework was intended to ensure a cautious and ethically justified application of PGT-M. However, it also created limitations when defining eligibility for adult-onset disorders, conditions with variable penetrance, and those with surveillance or preventive options.

HBOC exemplifies such a dilemma. Although carrying *BRCA1/2* pathogenic variants can lead to significant morbidity, their adult onset and the availability of surveillance and risk-reducing surgeries pose challenges to the current definition of severity.

4 Ethical and Social Considerations

Public and professional opinions on PGT-M have gradually shifted. Early discussions, especially in the 2000s, revealed strong resistance to PGT-M from both ethics committees and patient groups, largely due to fears of eugenics and discrimination. Amid growing recognition of diversity in society, however, by 2020, a shift toward recognizing individual reproductive autonomy was evident. Patients began to request PGT-M not out of rejection of affected individuals, but as a means to spare their children the hardships they themselves had experienced.

Nevertheless, tensions remain. Critics argue that PGT-M implies value judgments about lives worth living, particularly when conditions like HBOC are involved. Concerns have been raised about the social consequences of expanding PGT-M indications, such as increased pressure to undergo testing or marginalization of those with hereditary conditions.

5 Case Review and Committee Structures

Japan's approval process for PGT-M cases involves multiple layers of ethical and clinical review. Each application is evaluated based on the established eligibility criteria, often with input from clinical genetics experts, disease specialists, and patient support organizations. Recent changes allow couples to submit personal statements about how the disease affects their lives, providing a more holistic view.

For cases that do not fully meet the traditional severity criteria, the review now considers not only medical severity but also the couple's lived experiences and the human pain and suffering they have endured, allowing for a more comprehensive and individualized assessment. However, cases that clearly fall outside the framework are still reviewed but ultimately result in disapproval. This triage process has improved efficiency but continues to limit access for those affected by adult-onset or less penetrant diseases.

6 Challenges of HBOC and Adult-Onset Disorders

HBOC presents a unique challenge to the current framework. Despite the significant psychological and medical burden of *BRCA*-related cancers, JSOG has not yet approved PGT-M for HBOC cases as an indication. The availability of surveillance programs and preventive surgeries complicates the classification of HBOC as "untreatable" or "highly invasive," even though these interventions can be profoundly life-altering.

Surveys of both professionals and patients indicate divided opinions. While some argue that every couple deserves autonomy in reproductive decision-making, others caution against expanding PGT-M indications without societal consensus and robust ethical safeguards.

7 Expanding Perspectives and Future Directions

Discussions in recent JOHBOC meetings and working sessions suggest growing interest in reconsidering the parameters for determining eligibility. The rise of patient voices, growing acceptance of diversity in reproductive choices, and increasing awareness of psychological well-being all support a broader, more flexible framework.

Internationally, some guidelines have begun to incorporate broader definitions, acknowledging adult-onset conditions under specific circumstances. Japan may similarly benefit from adopting a multidimensional model that considers emotional burden, family context, and quality of life in assessing clinical seriousness.

8 Conclusion

The discussion around indications for PGT-M in Japan reflects a complex interplay of ethics, policy, medicine, and lived experience. While the current framework has ensured cautious and equitable implementation, there is increasing recognition that a more inclusive, patient-centered approach is needed. HBOC exemplifies the challenges and opportunities in evolving PGT-M policy. As societal values shift and reproductive medicine advances, Japan's definition of severity and eligibility for PGT-M must continue to adapt. This evolution should aim to balance scientific responsibility with reproductive autonomy.

References

1. Japan Society of Obstetrics and Gynecology. Statement on "pre-implantation diagnosis". J Japan Soc Obstet Gynecol. 1999;51(1):16–43. (in Japanese)
2. Committee on Ethics, Subcommittee on Preimplantation Diagnosis, Japan Society of Obstetrics and Gynecology. Report on the approval status and performance outcomes of preimplantation diagnosis (1999–2015). J Japan Soc Obstet Gynecol. 2017;69(9):1916–20. (in Japanese).
3. Japan Society of Obstetrics and Gynecology. Statement on "Pre-implantation Genetic Testing for Severe Genetic Diseases". 2022;74(3):363–70. (in Japanese)

Excellent General Presentation

Knock-In Rat Model of the BRCA1 Pathogenic Variant p.L63X: Its Basic Phenotypes and Perspectives for Use in Cancer Prevention Research

Tatsuhiko Imaoka, Yuzuki Nakamura, Kento Nagata, Yukiko Nishimura-Yano, Kazuhiro Daino, and Atsuko Ishikawa

Abstract Animal models are key to obtaining insights into disease mechanisms and developing prophylactic and treatment measures. We have recently developed a rat model of BRCA1 deficiency and revealed that this model mimics many of the phenotypes in humans. Herein, we briefly review the development and characterization of the phenotypes of this model.

T. Imaoka (✉)
Department of Radiation Effects Research, Institute for Radiological Science, National Institutes for Quantum Science and Technology (QST), Chiba, Japan

Institute for Quantum Life Science, National Institutes for Quantum Science and Technology (QST), Chiba, Japan

Department of Radiological Sciences, Graduate School of Human Health Sciences, Tokyo Metropolitan University, Tokyo, Japan
e-mail: imaoka.tatsuhiko@qst.go.jp

Y. Nakamura
Department of Radiation Effects Research, Institute for Radiological Science, National Institutes for Quantum Science and Technology (QST), Chiba, Japan

Department of Radiological Sciences, Graduate School of Human Health Sciences, Tokyo Metropolitan University, Arakawa-ku, Tokyo, Japan
e-mail: nakamura.yuzuki@qst.go.jp

K. Nagata · K. Daino
Department of Radiation Effects Research, Institute for Radiological Science, National Institutes for Quantum Science and Technology (QST), Chiba, Japan

Institute for Quantum Life Science, National Institutes for Quantum Science and Technology (QST), Chiba, Japan
e-mail: nagata.kento@qst.go.jp; daino.kazuhiro@qst.go.jp

Y. Nishimura-Yano · A. Ishikawa
Department of Radiation Effects Research, Institute for Radiological Science, National Institutes for Quantum Science and Technology (QST), Chiba, Japan
e-mail: nishimura.yukiko@qst.go.jp; ishikawa.atsuko@qst.go.jp

M. Arai et al. (eds.), *Practical Guide to Hereditary Breast and Ovarian Cancer IV*,
https://doi.org/10.1007/978-981-95-6580-1_21

Keywords Animal model · BRCA1 · Breast cancer · Hereditary breast and ovarian cancer · Radiation · Rat

1 Introduction

Hereditary breast and ovarian cancer (HBOC) is primarily associated with pathogenic variants of the *BRCA1* and *BRCA2* genes, which significantly increase the cancer risk of breast, ovary, biliary tract, esophagus, stomach, pancreas, and prostate [11]. One of the major clinical challenges in managing HBOC is early detection and prevention of cancer. Genetic testing and surveillance strategies help in early detection, but they do not prevent cancer development. Risk-reducing surgeries are effective but come with significant physical, emotional, and other quality-of-life consequences. Given these challenges, there is a growing need for chemoprevention, which involves using medications to reduce cancer risk. Selective estrogen receptor modulators have shown promise in reducing breast cancer risk in BRCA2 pathogenic variant carriers, and a recent analysis has supported a similar efficacy in BRCA1 pathogenic variant carriers [1]. However, it is not clear whether the efficacy of these drugs balances with their disadvantage.

The development of alternative chemoprevention strategies is thus warranted, and basic research—including studies using animal models—will be essential for uncovering safer and more effective preventive approaches. The authors recently reported on the development of a *Brca1* knock-in rat model [12]. Herein, we describe the development and characterization of this new rat model and review relevant studies.

2 Rationale for Developing Brca1-Deficient Rat Model

Animal models play a vital role in studying disease mechanisms and advancing treatment and prevention strategies. To date, researchers have developed over ten different animal models carrying *Brca1* mutations. While humans with heterozygous *BRCA1* pathogenic variants exhibit an increased risk of spontaneous breast cancer development, this phenomenon is not observed in heterozygous *Brca1* mutant mice [3–5]. Since mice with homozygous *Brca1* mutations do not survive, scientists have created conditional knockout models where the gene is selectively deleted in the mammary gland. Alternatively, for *Brca1* heterozygous mice, additional loss of one *Trp53* allele is necessary to significantly elevate mammary tumor formation. Consequently, these models may not fully capture the earliest stages of breast cancer development in individuals carrying *BRCA1* pathogenic variants.

While most unmodified mouse strains exhibit a low spontaneous incidence of mammary tumors, rats have historically served as an alternative model due to their ability to mimic the ductal and luminal characteristics of human breast cancer. Gene expression profiling has also indicated the relevance of rat models to human breast cancer [14]. Genetic modifications in rats were once difficult, but a groundbreaking study introduced a mutagenesis and screening approach that led to the development of the first *Brca1* knockout rat on a Sprague-Dawley background, a strain known for its high susceptibility to mammary cancer [21]. This rat model carries an intronic point mutation, which results in the loss of the last two exons, yet it did not exhibit an increased mammary tumor formation [17]. More recently, advancements in genome editing technologies have facilitated the creation of genetically engineered rat models.

3 Reported Phenotypes of *Brca1*$^{\text{p.L63X}}$ Knock-In Rats

3.1 *Embryonic Lethality of Homozygotes*

We chose to create a knock-in rat of the pathogenic variant p.L63X (hereafter L63X), a founder mutation frequently observed in Japan. Inheritance of the *Brca1*$^{\text{L63X}}$ allele was examined in offspring from four *Brca1*$^{\text{L63X/+}}$ female-male pairs. Allele-specific quantitative PCR analysis revealed the absence of *Brca1*$^{\text{L63X/L63X}}$ homozygotes, deviating significantly from Mendelian inheritance. Examination of pregnant uteri showed malformed conceptuses at mid-pregnancy, suggesting embryonic lethality. In contrast, *Brca1*$^{\text{L63X/+}}$ heterozygotes exhibited normal postnatal development, as indicated by body weight, organ size, and mammary gland morphology [12].

3.2 *Breast Cancer Phenotypes*

3.2.1 Spontaneous Cancer

To study spontaneous and induced mammary carcinogenesis, *Brca1*$^{\text{L63X/+}}$ and *Brca1*$^{+/+}$ rats were observed under untreated conditions. Ovarian cancers of epithelial origin, commonly seen in human HBOC patients, were not detected. Comparison of untreated *Brca1*$^{\text{L63X/+}}$ and *Brca1*$^{+/+}$ rats showed no significant difference in mammary cancer incidence. Histological analysis revealed no major differences between mammary tumors in *Brca1*$^{\text{L63X/+}}$ and *Brca1*$^{+/+}$ rats, but spontaneous carcinomas in *Brca1*$^{\text{L63X/+}}$ rats had a lower estrogen receptor α-positive cell fraction [12].

3.2.2 Chemically Induced Cancer

To investigate chemically induced carcinogenesis, rats were exposed to 25 or 50 mg/kg of 1-methyl-1-nitrosourea (MNU), a chemical carcinogen that forms methylated nucleotides such as O^6-methylguanine. MNU increased mammary cancer incidence in a dose-dependent manner, but differences between *Brca1*$^{L63X/+}$ and *Brca1*$^{+/+}$ rats were not statistically significant [12]. This result is plausible considering that MNU-induced DNA damage is repaired by other systems than homologous recombination repair, in which BRCA1 is involved.

3.2.3 Radiation-Induced Cancer

Radiation is known to produce DNA double-strand breaks in cells. The radiation risk in HBOC patients is especially relevant since some studies imply radiation-related risk of breast cancer in these patients [15, 19]. Radiation exposure during the postpubertal development showed a dose-dependent increase in mammary cancer incidence, with positive slopes in both genotypes of rats. Early-onset mammary cancer (i.e., that developing <40 weeks of age) was dose-dependent regardless of genotype, whereas middle-age cancer (i.e., that developing during 40–80 weeks of age) was significantly increased only in *Brca1*$^{L63X/+}$ rats. This result indicated a rather mild effect of the *Brca1* mutation. Since postpubertal radiation exposure is known to induce high breast cancer incidence in general [2, 6], we reasoned that the strong effect of the exposure may have masked the influence of *Brca1* mutation. Indeed, irradiation of prepubertal rats, which leads to a smaller mammary cancer increase in wild-type rats, resulted in significantly higher mammary cancer incidence in *Brca1*$^{L63X/+}$ rats than in *Brca1*$^{+/+}$ rats. Further investigation confirmed that loss of heterozygosity (LOH) at the *Brca1* locus was not involved in tumor development, and sequencing identified only minor somatic mutations, suggesting a non-mutational mechanism driving carcinogenesis in *Brca1*$^{L63X/+}$ rats [12].

The fact that *Brca1*$^{L63X/+}$ rats show breast cancer phenotype only after radiation exposure, with no indication of susceptibility to spontaneous or chemically induced carcinogenesis, implies that generation of DNA double-strand breaks by endogenous factors is a key mechanism in the breast cancer pathogenesis in humans. The retention of the wild-type allele in mammary cancer of *Brca1*$^{L63X/+}$ rats supports the role of BRCA1 haploinsufficiency [10].

3.3 *Oxidative-Stress-Induced Cancer Phenotypes*

3.3.1 Kidney Cancer

The control of oxidative stress is one of the multifaceted roles of BRCA1 [20]. Kong et al. [8] used male *Brca1*$^{L63X/+}$ rats to investigate oxidative stress-induced renal carcinogenesis via ferric nitrilotriacetate exposure. The mutant rats showed a significant increase in renal cell carcinoma incidence, with chromosomal amplifications resembling those seen in *BRCA1*-related breast cancers, including c-Myc amplification. An analysis of early changes in the kidney revealed iron metabolism dysregulation, mitochondrial malfunction, and renal tubular proliferation with iron overload. These findings suggest that biallelic wild-type *Brca1* protects mitochondrial metabolism under oxidative stress, preventing tumor development. Excess iron-driven oxidative stress may be a key driver of carcinogenesis in BRCA1 haploinsufficiency, offering potential targets for cancer prevention and therapy.

3.3.2 Malignant Mesothelioma

Malignant mesothelioma remains a major health concern linked to asbestos exposure, with local iron accumulation playing a central role in its pathogenesis. Luo et al. [9] used the *Brca1*$^{L63X/+}$ rats to demonstrate a promotional effect on mesothelial carcinogenesis in males exposed to chrysotile asbestos, but not crocidolite. Comparative genomic analysis of mesothelioma in mutant rats revealed more chromosomal deletions, including *Cdkn2a*/*Cdkn2b* loss and *Tfr2* amplification, alongside iron metabolism dysregulation. Mutant tumors exhibited ferroptosis resistance, characterized by increased *Slc7a11* and *Gpx4* expression. An analysis of early changes showed suppressed Brca1 expression in chrysotile-exposed mutants, implying that chrysotile asbestos poses a higher mesothelioma risk also in men harboring *BRCA1* pathogenic variants.

3.4 *Thyroid Tumors*

Nakamura et al. [13] backcrossed the *Brca1*$^{L63X/+}$ rats more than 12 times on the LEW background, which imposes less susceptibility to mammary carcinogenesis and moderate susceptibility to thyroid neoplasms. While the incidence of mammary cancer was similar between these *Brca1*$^{L63X/+}$ and *Brca1*$^{+/+}$ rats, either untreated or exposed to 2 Gy of γ rays, untreated *Brca1*$^{L63X/+}$ rats showed significantly higher prevalence of thyroid tumors than *Brca1*$^{+/+}$ rats. The *Brca1*$^{+/+}$ rats showed a tendency for increased prevalence of thyroid carcinoma after radiation exposure, but the prevalence did not differ between irradiated *Brca1*$^{L63X/+}$ and *Brca1*$^{+/+}$ rats. This finding implies a possible role of *BRCA1* pathogenic variants in the reported association between breast cancer family history and thyroid cancer risk [18, 22].

3.5 *Reproductive Phenotypes*

There is a noticeable pattern of diminished reproductive capacity in young, healthy women affected by HBOC syndrome, especially among those with *BRCA1* pathogenic variants [16]. Kaseki et al. [7] found reduced primordial follicle numbers accompanying age-related subfertility in *Brca1*$^{L63X/+}$ rats. Granulosa cells in young mutants exhibited elevated oxidative stress, with increased mTOR and decreased PTEN signaling. Treatment with olaparib, a poly(ADP-ribose) polymerase

Table 1 Phenotypes in *Brca1*$^{L63X/+}$ rats

Tissue	Phenotype	Reference
Fetus	Normal (embryonic lethality in homozygotes)	Nakamura et al. [12]
Breast (female)	Tumors having low ERα; unaltered spontaneous cancer incidence; unaltered cancer incidence after MNU exposure; increased cancer incidence after radiation exposure in some conditions	Nakamura et al. [12]
Thyroid (female)	High prevalence of tumors on the LEW background	Nakamura et al. [13]
Kidney (male)	High incidence of cancer after ferric nitrilotriacetate exposure	Kong et al. [8]
Mesothelium (male)	High incidence of cancer after chrysotile (but not crocidolite) asbestos exposure	Luo et al. [9]
Ovary	Reduced ovarian reserve; increased sensitivity to chemotherapeutics	Kaseki et al. [7]

inhibitor, further depleted primordial follicles, with upregulated DNA repair pathways. Combined olaparib and cyclophosphamide treatment led to severe ovarian toxicity, eliminating primordial follicles and inducing oocyte death via accumulated DNA damage. These findings highlight the need for reproductive consultation before chemotherapy in *BRCA1* pathogenic variant carriers, emphasizing the importance of evaluating ovarian reserve.

4 Conclusions

The reported phenotypes of the *Brca1*$^{L63X/+}$ rat model, as summarized in Table 1, indicate its usefulness in elucidating the molecular mechanisms of relevant pathogenesis and, potentially, strategic development of prophylactic measures.

Acknowledgements During the preparation of this work, the authors used an AI tool, Copilot (Microsoft), to enhance readability and language, aiding in formulating and structuring content. After using this tool, the authors reviewed and edited the content as needed and take full responsibility for the content of the publication.

References

1. Alwashmi ASS, Khan NU, Chen T. Risk-benefits assessment of tamoxifen or raloxifene as chemoprevention for risk reduction of breast cancer among BRCA1 and BRCA2 carriers: a meta-analysis. Sci Rep. 2025;15(1):6796. https://doi.org/10.1038/s41598-025-89915-z.
2. Brenner AV, Preston DL, Sakata R, Sugiyama H, de Gonzalez AB, French B, Utada M, Cahoon EK, Sadakane A, Ozasa K, Grant EJ, Mabuchi K. Incidence of breast cancer in the life span

study of atomic bomb survivors: 1958–2009. Radiat Res. 2018;190(4):433–44. https://doi.org/10.1667/RR15015.1.
3. Diaz-Cruz ES, Cabrera MC, Nakles R, Rutstein BH, Furth PA. BRCA1 deficient mouse models to study pathogenesis and therapy of triple negative breast cancer. Breast Dis. 2010;32(1–2):85–97. https://doi.org/10.3233/BD-2010-0308.
4. Drost RM, Jonkers J. Preclinical mouse models for BRCA1-associated breast cancer. Br J Cancer. 2009;101(10):1651–7. https://doi.org/10.1038/sj.bjc.6605350.
5. Evers B, Jonkers J. Mouse models of BRCA1 and BRCA2 deficiency: past lessons, current understanding and future prospects. Oncogene. 2006;25(43):5885–97. https://doi.org/10.1038/sj.onc.1209871.
6. Imaoka T, Nishimura M, Daino K, Kakinuma S. Modifiers of radiation effects on breast cancer incidence revealed by a reanalysis of archival data of rat experiments. J Radiat Res. 2023;64(2):273–83. https://doi.org/10.1093/jrr/rrac090.
7. Kaseki S, Sonehara R, Motooka Y, Tanaka H, Nakamura T, Osuka S, Akatsuka S, Kajiyama H, Mashimo T, Imaoka T, Toyokuni S. Susceptibility of Brca1((L63X/+)) rat to ovarian reserve dissipation by chemotherapeutic agents to breast cancer. Cancer Sci. 2025;116(4):1139–52. https://doi.org/10.1111/cas.16412.
8. Kong Y, Akatsuka S, Motooka Y, Zheng H, Cheng Z, Shiraki Y, Mashimo T, Imaoka T, Toyokuni S. BRCA1 haploinsufficiency promotes chromosomal amplification under Fenton reaction-based carcinogenesis through ferroptosis-resistance. Redox Biol. 2022;54:102356. https://doi.org/10.1016/j.redox.2022.102356.
9. Luo Y, Akatsuka S, Motooka Y, Kong Y, Zheng H, Mashimo T, Imaoka T, Toyokuni S. BRCA1 haploinsufficiency impairs iron metabolism to promote chrysotile-induced mesothelioma via ferroptosis resistance. Cancer Sci. 2023;114(4):1423–36. https://doi.org/10.1111/cas.15705.
10. Minello A, Carreira A. BRCA1/2 Haploinsufficiency: exploring the impact of losing one allele. J Mol Biol. 2024;436(1):168277. https://doi.org/10.1016/j.jmb.2023.168277.
11. Momozawa Y, Iwasaki Y, Parsons MT, Kamatani Y, Takahashi A, Tamura C, Katagiri T, Yoshida T, Nakamura S, Sugano K, Miki Y, Hirata M, Matsuda K, Spurdle AB, Kubo M. Germline pathogenic variants of 11 breast cancer genes in 7,051 Japanese patients and 11,241 controls. Nat Commun. 2018;9(1):4083. https://doi.org/10.1038/s41467-018-06581-8.
12. Nakamura Y, Kubota J, Nishimura Y, Nagata K, Nishimura M, Daino K, Ishikawa A, Kaneko T, Mashimo T, Kokubo T, Takabatake M, Inoue K, Fukushi M, Arai M, Saito M, Shimada Y, Kakinuma S, Imaoka T. *Brca1*$^{L63X/+}$ rat is a novel model of human BRCA1 deficiency displaying susceptibility to radiation-induced mammary cancer. Cancer Sci. 2022;113(10):3362–73. https://doi.org/10.1111/cas.15485.
13. Nakamura Y, Nishimura-Yano Y, Nishimura M, Kokubo T, Daino K, Takabatake M, Nagata K, Mashimo T, Kakinuma S, Inoue K, Imaoka T. Spontaneous and radiation-induced mammary and thyroid tumorigenesis in LEW and (SD×COP)F_1*Brca1*$^{L63X/+}$ rats. Anticancer Res. 2025;45(11):4869–80. https://doi.org/10.21873/anticanres.17834.
14. Nishimura Y, Iizuka D, Takabatake M, Daino K, Nishimura M, Morioka T, Shimada Y, Kakinuma S, Imaoka T. Characterization of molecular subtypes of rat mammary cancer and their association with environmental exposures. Anticancer Res. 2024;44(10):4261–72. https://doi.org/10.21873/anticanres.17256.
15. Pijpe A, Andrieu N, Easton DF, Kesminiene A, Cardis E, Nogues C, Gauthier-Villars M, Lasset C, Fricker JP, Peock S, Frost D, Evans DG, Eeles RA, Paterson J, Manders P, van Asperen CJ, Ausems MG, Meijers-Heijboer H, Thierry-Chef I, Hauptmann M, Goldgar D, Rookus MA, van Leeuwen FE, Genepso E, Hebon. Exposure to diagnostic radiation and risk of breast cancer among carriers of BRCA1/2 mutations: retrospective cohort study (GENE-RAD-RISK). BMJ. 2012;345:e5660. https://doi.org/10.1136/bmj.e5660.
16. Sighinolfi G, Grandi G, Barbieri E, Venturelli M, Piombino C, Melotti C, Lippi Bruni R, Costantini Cuoghi R, D'Amico R, Lambertini M, Peccatori FA, Tenedini E, Dominici M, Cortesi L, La Marca A, Toss A. Reduced reproductive potential in young healthy women

with hereditary breast and/or ovarian cancer syndrome. Commun Med (Lond). 2025;5(1):70. https://doi.org/10.1038/s43856-025-00788-9.
17. Smits BM, Cotroneo MS, Haag JD, Gould MN. Genetically engineered rat models for breast cancer. Breast Dis. 2007;28:53–61. https://doi.org/10.3233/bd-2007-28106.
18. Song H, Jung YS, Tran TXM, Moon CM, Park B. Increased risk of pancreatic, thyroid, prostate and breast cancers in men with a family history of breast cancer: a population-based study. Int J Cancer. 2023;153(5):950–7. https://doi.org/10.1002/ijc.34573.
19. van Barele M, Akdeniz D, Heemskerk-Gerritsen BA, Genepso, Andrieu N, Nogues C, Hebon, van Asperen CJ, Wevers M, Ausems MG, de Bock GH. Contralateral breast cancer risk in patients with breast cancer and a germline-BRCA1/2 pathogenic variant undergoing radiation. J Natl Cancer Inst. 2023;115(11):1318–28. https://doi.org/10.1093/jnci/djad116.
20. Yi YW, Kang HJ, Bae I. BRCA1 and oxidative stress. Cancers (Basel). 2014;6(2):771–95. https://doi.org/10.3390/cancers6020771.
21. Zan Y, Haag JD, Chen KS, Shepel LA, Wigington D, Wang YR, Hu R, Lopez-Guajardo CC, Brose HL, Porter KI, Leonard RA, Hitt AA, Schommer SL, Elegbede AF, Gould MN. Production of knockout rats using ENU mutagenesis and a yeast-based screening assay. Nat Biotechnol. 2003;21(6):645–51. https://doi.org/10.1038/nbt830.
22. Zheng G, Yu H, Hemminki A, Forsti A, Sundquist K, Hemminki K. Familial associations of female breast cancer with other cancers. Int J Cancer. 2017;141(11):2253–9. https://doi.org/10.1002/ijc.30927.

Evaluation of BRCAness in Brain Metastasis Lesions of Breast Cancer Patients

Yumiko Ishizuka, Yoshiya Horimoto, Hidetaka Eguchi, Fumi Murakami, Junichiro Watanabe, and Masami Arai

Abstract Purpose: BRCAness is defined as the status of homologous recombination deficiency (HRD) in tumor tissue, regardless of the presence of pathogenic germline *BRCA1/2* variants. A study employing next-generation sequencing analysis showed that HRD was found relatively frequently in brain metastases of breast cancer patients. One of the methods to assess BRCAness is multiplex ligation-dependent probe amplification (MLPA) assay; however, there have been no studies evaluating BRCAness in brain metastases of breast cancer based on MLPA techniques.

Y. Ishizuka (✉) · F. Murakami · J. Watanabe
Department of Breast Oncology, Juntendo University Faculty of Medicine, Bunkyo-ku, Tokyo, Japan
e-mail: y-ishizuka@juntendo.ac.jp

Y. Horimoto
Department of Breast Oncology, Juntendo University Faculty of Medicine, Bunkyo-ku, Tokyo, Japan

Department of Human Pathology, Juntendo University Faculty of Medicine, Bunkyo-ku, Tokyo, Japan

Department of Breast Surgery and Oncology, Tokyo Medical University, Shinjuku-ku, Tokyo, Japan

H. Eguchi
Diagnostics and Therapeutics of Intractable Disease, Juntendo University Graduate School of Medicine, Bunkyo-ku, Tokyo, Japan

M. Arai
Department of Breast Oncology, Juntendo University Faculty of Medicine, Bunkyo-ku, Tokyo, Japan

Diagnostics and Therapeutics of Intractable Disease, Juntendo University Graduate School of Medicine, Bunkyo-ku, Tokyo, Japan

Clinical Genetics, Juntendo University Graduate School of Medicine, Bunkyo-ku, Tokyo, Japan

M. Arai et al. (eds.), *Practical Guide to Hereditary Breast and Ovarian Cancer IV*,
https://doi.org/10.1007/978-981-95-6580-1_22

Methods: We retrospectively investigated 15 brain metastases of breast cancer that were surgically resected at our hospital from January 2007 to December 2022. To evaluate BRCAness, we employed the MLPA method.

Results: Of the 15 patients, five patients (33%) had tumors with BRCAness. Clinicopathological factors of patients with brain metastases with BRCAness were not statistically different from those of patients who possessed tumors without BRCAness. Meanwhile, patients with brain metastases with BRCAness had shorter overall survival compared to those without BRCAness (P = 0.013, BRCAness: median 15 months (95% CI; 2–30) vs non-BRCAness: median 28.5 months (95% CI; 10–60)).

Conclusion: In this study, we evaluated BRCAness in brain metastases of breast cancer with the MLPA method and found that about one-third of patients had BRCAness-positive tumors.

Keywords Breast cancer · Brain metastasis · BRCAness · Homologous recombination deficiency (HRD) · Poly ADP-ribose polymerase inhibitors

1 Introduction

Breast cancer is one of the most common carcinomas to develop central nervous system (CNS) metastases, along with lung cancer [1]. The prognosis of patients with CNS metastases is poor [2–5]; for example, the median overall survival (OS) with breast cancer brain metastases (BCBM) was around 7–10 months. Although systemic therapy has been thought to be ineffective for BCBM in the past, newer agents are expected to be more effective [6, 7]. However, evidence of the therapeutic effects, particularly of therapies other than anti-HER2 drugs, is still lacking.

The status of homologous recombination deficiency (HRD) in tumor tissue is referred to as BRCAness, regardless of the presence or absence of pathogenic germline *BRCA1/2* variants [8]. HRD, including BRCA1/2 dysfunction, is expected to be a potential biomarker for Poly ADP-ribose polymerase (PARP) inhibitors (PARPi) therapy [9–11]. MyChoice Diagnostic System for assessing HRD in tumor tissues has also become available for breast cancer patients. Recently, a study using whole-exome sequencing analyses reported that HRD was found relatively frequently in BCBM [12]. There are several methods to assess BRCAness [13, 14]. To date, there have been no studies evaluating BRCAness in BM based on multiplex ligation-dependent probe amplification (MLPA) techniques. Therefore, in this study, we evaluated BRCAness in BM lesions of breast cancer patients employing the method.

2 Material and Methods

2.1 Clinical Samples

In total, 17 patients with BCBM underwent surgical resection at our hospital from January 2007 to December 2022. Of these, samples from 15 patients were able to be analyzed, while DNA from two samples did not meet the quality and quantity requirements for analysis. OS was defined as the length of time that the patient survived from the detection of BM.

2.2 BRCAness Evaluation

BRCAness was determined by MLPA, which is based on the characteristic copy number variations (CNVs) as determined by BRCA1-like array comparative genomic hybridization pattern. Classification of BRCAness subtypes was performed by MLPA with the P376-B4 BRCA1ness SALSA MLPA probe mix (MRC-Holland, Amsterdam, The Netherlands) as described previously [14, 15]. The BRCAness score was calculated with the relative copy number ratio obtained by comparing each sample with the reference sample. Following the manufacturer's protocol, a sample with a BRCAness score of ≥ 0.5 was classified as having BRCAness. If the score was <0.5, the sample was classified as not having BRCAness.

3 Results

3.1 Clinicopathological Findings

The clinicopathological features of the 15 cases assessed are shown in Table 1. All patients were Japanese women ranging in age from 43 to 75 years (median, 67 years) at the detection of BM. The median duration until BM after curative surgery for breast cancer was 32.5 months (range, 0–198 months). As to the subtype of BM, seven patients had luminal tumors, four patients had luminal-HER2 tumors, one patient had a HER2 tumor, and three patients had triple-negative (TN) tumors.

3.2 BRCAness Evaluation in Brain Metastases

Of the 15 patients, five patients (33%) had brain metastases with BRCAness. Among the five patients whose BM showed BRCAness, samples of primary breast cancer were available from four patients, and we analyzed these primary breast tumors for

Table 1 The Clinicopathological features of the 15 patients

Case no.	Age (*y*)	Time to BM[a] (*m*)	Subtype	BRCAness		
				BM	Primary tumor	Genetic testing for *BRCA1/2* genes
1	68	20	Luminal	BRCAness	BRCAness	N.E.
2	67	34	TN	BRCAness	N.E.	N.E.
3	67	34	TN	BRCAness	BRCAness	N.E.
4	75	198	Luminal-HER2	BRCAness	Non-BRCAness	N.E.
5	46	11	Luminal	BRCAness	BRCAness	No pathogenic variants
6	67	0[b]	Luminal	Non-BRCAness	N.E.	N.E.
7	70	139	Luminal	Non-BRCAness	N.E.	N.E.
8	58	31	HER	Non-BRCAness	N.E.	N.E.
9	61	123	Luminal	Non-BRCAness	N.E.	N.E.
10	47	27	Luminal-HER2	Non-BRCAness	N.E.	N.E.
11	45	26	Luminal-HER2	Non-BRCAness	N.E.	N.E.
12	43	34	Luminal	Non-BRCAness	N.E.	N.E.
13	72	Unknown	TN	Non-BRCAness	N.E.	N.E.
14	71	Unknown	Luminal-HER2	Non-BRCAness	N.E.	N.E.
15	75	Unknown	Luminal	Non-BRCAness	N.E.	N.E.

BM brain metastasis, *HER2* human epidermal growth factor receptor 2, *N.E.* not evaluated, *TN* triple negative

[a]Duration from the time of primary breast cancer diagnosis

[b]*De novo* stage IV

BRCAness. We found that three patients (75%, 3/4) had primary breast tumors with BRCAness. Among all 15 patients, only Case #5 had received genetic testing for the BRCA1/2 genes. No pathogenic germline variants in these genes were detected, while she had a primary breast tumor with BRCAness.

The comparison of clinicopathological features between patients with BRCAness ($n = 5$) and without BRCAness ($n = 10$) is shown in Table 2. There were no significant differences between groups in age, the number of other organs with metastases, ER and HER2 status, the number of regimens applied before BM diagnosis, and history of radiation therapy (RT) to the brain.

Table 2 Clinicopathological features according to BRCAness status

		BRCAness	Non-BRCAness	*P*-value
		n (%)	*n* (%)	
n		5	10	
Age, median (range), *y*		67.0 (46–75)	64.0 (43–75)	0.575
Period until BM, median (range), *m*		34.0 (11–198)	31.0 (0–139)	0.895
Number of extracranial lesions, median (range)		0 (0–1)	0.5 (0–3)	0.437
ER status	Positive	3 (60.0)	9 (90.0)	0.242
	Negative	2 (40.0)	1 (10.0)	
HER2 status	Positive	1 (20.0)	4 (40.0)	0.600
	Negative	4 (80.0)	6 (60.0)	
Number of regimens of previous	Chemotherapy	2.0 (1–3)	1.0 (0–3)	0.150
Systemic treatment until BM, median (range)	Anti-HER2 therapy	0	0 (0–1)	0.089
	Endocrine therapy	1.0 (0–1)	0 (0–1)	0.373
	Total	2.0 (2–3)	1.0 (0–4)	0.444
History of RT to brain		0	5 (50.0)	0.101

Values are *n* (%) unless otherwise indicated
BM brain metastasis, *ER* estrogen receptor, *HER2* human epidermal growth factor receptor 2, *RT* radiation therapy

3.3 Patient Outcomes

During the median 30-month observation period (range, 3–79 months), 11 patients (73.3%) died of breast cancer. We investigated the relationship between clinicopathological factors and OS. Univariate analysis revealed that BRCAness was related to OS ($P = 0.025$), i.e., patients with BRCAness had significantly shorter OS (BRCAness vs. non-BRCAness: median, 15 months vs. 28.5 months). There were no differences in other factors, such as age, the number of extracranial lesions, ER and HER2 status, and having received RT.

Finally, we drew Kaplan-Meier curves of OS according to BRCAness (Fig. 1). Patients with BRCAness had significantly shorter OS compared to patients without BRCAness ($P = 0.013$). No significant effect of prior brain radiation or the presence of extracranial metastases on OS was observed, supporting that BRCAness status itself was the main prognostic factor in this cohort.

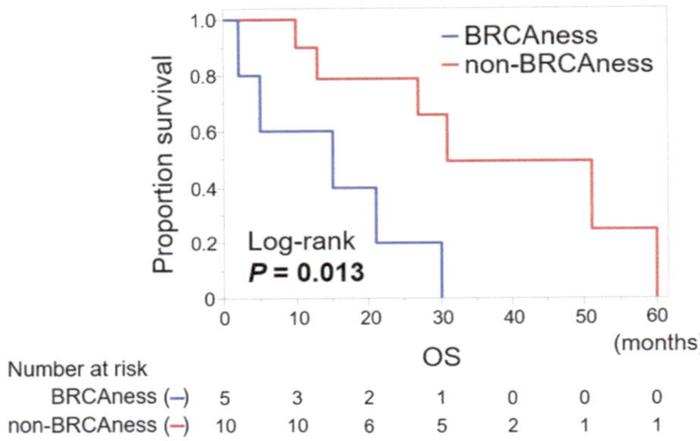

Fig. 1 Kaplan-Meier curves of overall survival (OS) according to the status of BRCAnessKaplan-Meier curves of OS from the detection of brain metastases according to the status of BRCAness are shown. Blue curves indicate patients with brain metastases with BRCAness, while red curves indicate patients with brain metastases without BRCAness

4 Discussion

In this study, we evaluated BRCAness in BM specimens in patients with metastatic breast cancer using the MLPA method, which is a relatively lower-cost, rapid, and simple procedure. To our knowledge, this is the first report to evaluate BRCAness in BCBM using this method. About one-third of patients with brain metastases had BRCAness. Patients with brain metastases with BRCAness had significantly shorter OS than those that did not display BRCAness, while clinicopathological factors of the patients did not differ between these two groups. And we found the BRCAness of the brain lesion affects patients' outcomes.

As for the causes of BRCAness in breast cancer patients besides genetic *BRCA1/2* mutations, the accumulation of somatic mutations of various genes is known to cause BRCAness [16]. Epigenetic factors, such as methylation of promoter regions, can also cause HRD [17]. In addition, systemic treatments might also have an impact on BRCAness developing. Furthermore, the disease progression of breast cancer may induce BRCAness. Diossy et al. reported that developing HRD in BM required a relatively long time [12].

In conclusion, a certain proportion of BCBM showed BRCAness, which could be evaluated by the MLPA method. Since BRCAness may be enhanced in metastatic lesions, evaluating BRCAness in metastatic lesions is of particular importance. It remains unclear whether this phenomenon is specific to brain metastases, and further studies investigating other metastatic sites are warranted. Moreover, assessing the therapeutic efficacy of PARP inhibitors in tumors exhibiting BRCAness will be an important future direction. To elucidate the mechanism of BRCAness, it is expected that more research will be done including BRCAness at other metastasis sites.

This manuscript is based on our study published in 2023 [18] and later presented at the Annual Meeting of the Japanese Organization of Hereditary Breast and Ovarian Cancer 2024.

References

1. Eichler AF, Loeffler JS. Multidisciplinary management of brain metastases. Oncologist. 2007;12:884–98.
2. Niikura N, Hayashi N, Masuda N, et al. Treatment outcomes and prognostic factors for patients with brain metastases from breast cancer of each subtype: a multicenter retrospective analysis. Breast Cancer Res Treat. 2014;147:103–12.
3. Darlix A, Louvel G, Fraisse J, et al. Impact of breast cancer molecular subtypes on the incidence, kinetics and prognosis of central nervous system metastases in a large multicentre real-life cohort. Br J Cancer. 2019;121:991–1000.
4. Matsuo S, Watanabe J, Mitsuya K, et al. Brain metastasis in patients with metastatic breast cancer in the real world: a single-institution, retrospective review of 12-year follow-up. Breast Cancer Res Treat. 2017;162:169–79.
5. Watanabe J, Mitsuya K, Nakamoto S, et al. Leptomeningeal metastasis in ER+HER2-advanced breast cancer patients: a review of the cases in a single institute over a 15-year period. Breast Cancer Res Treat. 2021;189:225–36.
6. Bailleux C, Eberst L, Bachelot T. Treatment strategies for breast cancer brain metastases. Br J Cancer. 2021;124:142–55.
7. Watase C, Shiino S, Shimoi T, et al. Breast cancer brain metastasis-overview of disease state, treatment options and future perspectives. Cancers (Basel). 2021;13(5):1078. https://doi.org/10.3390/cancers13051078.
8. Turner N, Tutt A, Ashworth A. Hallmarks of 'BRCAness' in sporadic cancers. Nat Rev Cancer. 2004;4:814–9.
9. Severson TM, Wolf DM, Yau C, et al. The BRCA1ness signature is associated significantly with response to PARP inhibitor treatment versus control in the I-SPY 2 randomized neoadjuvant setting. Breast Cancer Res. 2017;19:99.
10. Abbotts R, Dellomo AJ, Rassool FV. Pharmacologic induction of BRCAness in BRCA-proficient cancers: expanding PARP inhibitor use. Cancers (Basel). 2022;14:2640.
11. Oshi M, Gandhi S, Wu R, et al. Development of a novel BRCAness score that predicts response to PARP inhibitors. Biomark Res. 2022;10:80.
12. Diossy M, Reiniger L, Sztupinszki Z, et al. Breast cancer brain metastases show increased levels of genomic aberration-based homologous recombination deficiency scores relative to their corresponding primary tumors. Ann Oncol. 2018;29:1948–54.
13. Vollebergh MA, Lips EH, Nederlof PM, et al. An aCGH classifier derived from BRCA1-mutated breast cancer and benefit of high-dose platinum-based chemotherapy in HER2-negative breast cancer patients. Ann Oncol. 2011;22:1561–70.
14. Lips EH, Laddach N, Savola SP, et al. Quantitative copy number analysis by Multiplex Ligation-dependent Probe Amplification (MLPA) of BRCA1-associated breast cancer regions identifies BRCAness. Breast Cancer Res. 2011;13:R107.
15. Joosse SA, van Beers EH, Tielen IH, et al. Prediction of BRCA1-association in hereditary non-BRCA1/2 breast carcinomas with array-CGH. Breast Cancer Res Treat. 2009;116:479–89.
16. Lord CJ, Ashworth A. BRCAness revisited. Nat Rev Cancer. 2016;16:110–20.
17. Polak P, Kim J, Braunstein LZ, et al. A mutational signature reveals alterations underlying deficient homologous recombination repair in breast cancer. Nat Genet. 2017;49:1476–86.
18. Ishizuka Y, Horimoto Y, Eguchi H, et al. BRCAness of brain lesions reflects a worse outcome for patients with metastatic breast cancer. Breast Cancer Res Treat. 2024;203:49–55.

BRCA2 c.7847C>T (p.Ser2616Phe): A Pathogenic Variant Specific to the Japanese Population

Kazuki Yamazawa

Abstract Variants of uncertain significance (VUS) in *BRCA1/2* remain a persistent challenge for clinical genetics because they complicate genetic counseling and may limit access to targeted therapies. The *BRCA2* c.7847C>T (p.Ser2616Phe) variant recurs almost exclusively among Japanese individuals and has been reported as a VUS. Integrating nationwide registry data, clinic-based ascertainment, literature review, and orthogonal functional genomics, the totality of evidence now supports reclassification to likely pathogenic. Carriers present ages at first cancer onset, histopathology, and tumor spectra compatible with *BRCA2*-associated hereditary breast and ovarian cancer (HBOC). Population resources demonstrate absence from large global datasets and extremely low frequency in Japanese reference panels, consistent with a rare, population-specific variant. Quantitative co-segregation from informative pedigrees was not conclusive due to a limited number of genotyped individuals; however, the evidence becomes more convincing when combined with high-throughput functional assays demonstrating deleterious effects consistent with *BRCA2* loss-of-function. According to the American College of Medical Genetics and Genomics and the Association for Molecular Pathology (ACMG/AMP) guidelines, criteria PS3, PM2, and PM3 together with PP3 are met, justifying a likely pathogenic designation. These findings have implications for surveillance, cascade testing, and therapeutic decision-making in Japan.

Keywords BRCA2, Hereditary breast and ovarian cancer (HBOC) · American College of Medical Genetics and Genomics and the Association for Molecular Pathology (ACMG/AMP) guidelines · Variant of uncertain significance (VUS) · Reclassification · Founder variant

---

K. Yamazawa (✉)
Department of Medical Genetics, NHO Tokyo Medical Center, Tokyo, Japan
e-mail: kyamazawa@ntmc-genet.jp

M. Arai et al. (eds.), *Practical Guide to Hereditary Breast and Ovarian Cancer IV*,
https://doi.org/10.1007/978-981-95-6580-1_23

1 Introduction

The widespread clinical implementation of *BRCA1/2* genetic testing has transformed prevention, early detection, and treatment in HBOC, yet VUS remain a major obstacle to clinical application. Variants of uncertain significance (VUS) generate uncertainty for at-risk relatives, complicate decisions regarding risk-reducing surgery, and may preclude eligibility for poly(ADP-ribose) polymerase (PARP) inhibitors even in advanced disease [1]. In this context, certain VUS recur in specific populations, raising the possibility of founder effects and facilitating resolution through ancestry-aware analysis. The *BRCA2* c.7847C>T (p.Ser2616Phe) variant is a salient example: it has been observed in Japanese families while being essentially absent elsewhere [1], prompting a systematic effort to aggregate genetic, clinical, and functional evidence to determine its clinical significance. This chapter summarizes the integrated analysis that supports reclassification to likely pathogenic and highlights practical implications for clinical genetics in Japan.

2 Population and Genetic Evidence

Population frequency is a fundamental consideration in variant interpretation. At the time of the comprehensive analysis, the *BRCA2* c.7847C>T (p.Ser2616Phe) variant was absent from global population databases such as gnomAD and TOPMed and present at a very low allele frequency in ToMMo 38KJPN (8/77,444; 1.03×10^{-4}), indicating rarity even within Japanese controls [1]. Disease databases historically listed the variant as of uncertain significance, reflecting limited prior evidence and emphasizing the need for multifactorial assessment [1]. The geographic and ethnic distribution of observed carriers, restricted to Japan in clinical cohorts and literature, strongly suggests a population-specific variant with a plausible founder effect [1]. This ancestry-aware context increases the likelihood that the variant contributes to HBOC risk among Japanese families while remaining extremely rare in other populations.

3 Clinical Phenotype and Co-segregation

Across families ascertained through clinics, a national registry, and prior reports, carriers manifested breast and ovarian cancers with ages at first onset and histopathology compatible with *BRCA2*-associated HBOC [1]. Tumor types included luminal and triple-negative breast cancers as well as high-grade serous ovarian carcinoma. Quantitative co-segregation analysis was attempted but not conclusive because only a limited number of relatives were available for genotyping in each family [1].

Within the ACMG/AMP framework, such limitations underscore the value of orthogonal functional assays to complement segregation data [2].

4 Functional Evidence from Validated Assays

Functional genomics provided pivotal evidence for classification. Using *BRCA2*-deficient human cells and selective pressure with a PARP inhibitor, the MANO-B assay quantified variant-specific effects. Benchmarking of the MANO-B assay has demonstrated high sensitivity and specificity in distinguishing pathogenic from benign variants, supporting its use as strong functional evidence [3]. According to the MANO-B assay, the c.7847C>T (p.Ser2616Phe) variant was categorized as fClass 5 (pathogenic) [1] (Fig. 1).

5 Additional Supporting Observations

Orthogonal lines of evidence reinforce the functional findings. In a Japanese Fanconi anemia patient, an autosomal recessive condition requiring biallelic *BRCA2* loss-of-function, c.7847C>T was observed *in trans* with a known pathogenic *BRCA2* splice variant (c.475+1G>A), supporting application of PM3 [4]. In silico predictors converge on deleteriousness and conservation analyses disfavor phenylalanine at residue 2616; for example, the reported CADD score was 27.0, with PolyPhen-2 “probably damaging,” SIFT “damaging,” and MutationTaster “disease causing” [1].

6 Integrated Classification Under the ACMG/AMP Guidelines

Applying the ACMG/AMP guidelines yields a transparent classification. PS3 is satisfied based on validated functional assays demonstrating loss-of-function; PM2 is met by absence from global datasets together with extreme rarity in Japanese controls; PM3 is supported by the trans configuration with a pathogenic *BRCA2* variant in a Fanconi anemia case; PP3 is met through concordant deleterious computational predictions. PP4 was not invoked because carriers’ tumor spectra align with the *BRCA2* phenotype rather than a syndrome uniquely specific to this variant. Altogether, the *BRCA2* c.7847C>T (p.Ser2616Phe) variant is classified as likely pathogenic.

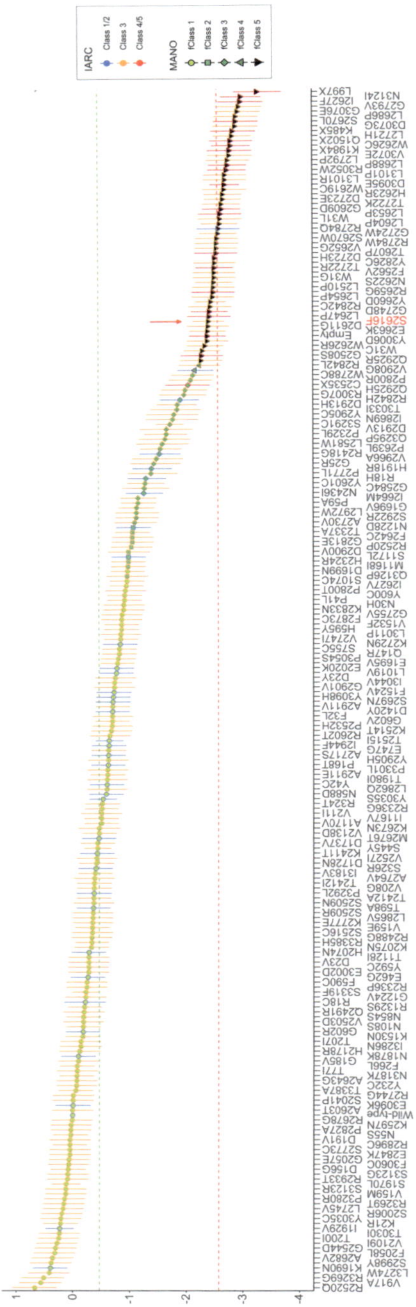

Fig. 1 Evaluation of the *BRCA2* c.7847C>T (p.Ser2616Phe) variant and other 244 variants by the MANO-B method. Bar plots of functional variant effects and functional diagnosis of the *BRCA2* c.7847C>T (p.Ser2616Phe) variant as well as other 244 *BRCA2* variants, sorted by a variant-specific effect value, *η*. The upper (green) and lower (red) dotted lines indicate the median values of normal-function and loss-of-function components, respectively. The categorization of each variant based on the IARC classification and the Bayes factor obtained by the MANO-B assay is indicated by the color and shape of the lines and plots, as shown in the legend. *N* = 3 cells were examined over 3 independent experimental batches. Plots indicate mean values, and open error bars indicate 95% confidence intervals. The variant-specific effect of c.7847C>T (p.Ser2616Phe) is depicted by a red arrow and highlighted in red. (Reproduced from Yamazawa et al. [1], with permission. © The Authors. Licensed under CC BY-NC 4.0)

7 Clinical Implications for Practice in Japan

A likely pathogenic designation has immediate implications. Risk assessment and surveillance should follow recommendations for *BRCA2* pathogenic-variant carriers, with intensified screening and consideration of risk-reducing procedures based on age and family history. Cascade testing among at-risk relatives is a priority; the plausible founder effect implies that identifying one carrier may uncover additional relatives who can benefit from surveillance and prevention. In oncology, classification as likely pathogenic may inform consideration of platinum-based chemotherapy and PARP inhibitors in appropriate clinical contexts characterized by homologous recombination deficiency, consistent with the companion-diagnostic role discussed for the MANO-B assay [3].

8 Operational Considerations for Laboratories and Expert Panels

From a laboratory standpoint, curation should clearly describe how each piece of evidence maps to specific ACMG/AMP criteria, so that users can review the reasoning and update classifications as new data become available [2, 5, 6]. The MANO-B functional results should be highlighted explicitly, while segregation analyses should include clear statements of assumptions and provide summaries of pedigrees. Population data should be stratified by ancestry, given that this variant is largely restricted to Japanese cohorts. Finally, submissions to ClinVar and national databases should be updated to indicate a likely pathogenic classification, using harmonized wording across institutions to reduce conflicting interpretations [2, 6].

9 Future Directions

Three points warrant emphasis. First, haplotype analysis across independent carrier families would directly test the founder hypothesis. Second, expanded family studies, particularly in pedigrees with multiple affected individuals, would strengthen segregation evidence. Third, prospective clinical registries capturing penetrance, age-specific risks, and therapy responses among carriers will refine counseling and treatment in Japan [1].

10 Conclusions

The accumulated genetic, clinical, and functional evidence supports reclassification of the *BRCA2* c.7847C>T (p.Ser2616Phe) variant from VUS to likely pathogenic in the Japanese population. The variant is absent from global cohorts and extremely rare in Japanese controls, and it recurs across unrelated Japanese families. Validated functional assays provide strong evidence of loss of function, while segregation and computational analyses add convergent support. According to the ACMG/AMP guidelines, PS3, PM2, PM3, and PP3 are met, yielding a clinically meaningful classification that enables more confident counseling, surveillance, cascade testing, and therapeutic considerations in Japan [1].

References

1. Yamazawa K, Sugano K, Tanakaya K, et al. The pathogenic role of the BRCA2 c.7847C>T (p.Ser2616Phe) variant in breast and ovarian cancer predisposition. Cancer Sci. 2023;114(7):2993–3002. https://doi.org/10.1111/cas.15799.
2. Richards S, Aziz N, Bale S, et al. Standards and guidelines for the interpretation of sequence variants: a joint consensus recommendation of the American College of Medical Genetics and Genomics and the Association for Molecular Pathology. Genet Med. 2015;17(5):405–24. https://doi.org/10.1038/gim.2015.30.
3. Ikegami M, Kohsaka S, Ueno T, et al. High-throughput functional evaluation of BRCA2 variants of unknown significance. Nat Commun. 2020;11(1):2573. https://doi.org/10.1038/s41467-020-16141-8.
4. Mori M, Hira A, Yoshida K, et al. Pathogenic mutations identified by a multimodality approach in 117 Japanese Fanconi anemia patients. Haematologica. 2019;104(10):1962–73. https://doi.org/10.3324/haematol.2018.207241.
5. Tavtigian SV, Greenblatt MS, Harrison SM, et al. Modeling the ACMG/AMP variant classification guidelines as a Bayesian classification framework. Genet Med. 2018;20(9):1054–60. https://doi.org/10.1038/gim.2017.210.
6. Brnich SE, Abou Tayoun AN, Couch FJ, et al. Recommendations for application of the functional evidence PS3/BS3 criterion using the ACMG/AMP sequence variant interpretation framework. Genome Med. 2019;12(1):3. https://doi.org/10.1186/s13073-019-0690-2.

Prevalence and Characteristics of Pathogenic Variants in BRCA1/2 Genes in the Japanese Population

Tasuku Mariya, Masashi Idogawa, Tsuyoshi Saito, Hiroshi Nakase, and Akihiro Sakurai

Abstract The content we presented at the Annual Meeting of the Japanese Organization of Hereditary Breast and Ovarian Cancer 2024 was based on an investigation into how many carriers of pathogenic *BRCA1/2* variants (i.e., individuals with HBOC) are included in ToMMo-54KJPN, the standard Japanese genome reference panel. Remarkably, the frequency of individuals harboring pathogenic variants in either *BRCA1* or *BRCA2* reached 5.772×10^{-3}, which was considerably higher than anticipated. Furthermore, by comparing the ranking of variant frequencies in

T. Mariya (✉)
Division of Clinical Genomics, Department of Genomic and Preventive Medicine, Sapporo Medical University School of Medicine, Sapporo, Japan

Department of Obstetrics and Gynecology, Sapporo Medical University School of Medicine, Sapporo, Japan
e-mail: mariya.tasuku@sapmed.ac.jp

M. Idogawa
Division of Medical Genome Sciences, Department of Genomic and Preventive Medicine, Sapporo Medical University School of Medicine, Sapporo, Japan

Department of Gastroenterology and Hepatology, Sapporo Medical University School of Medicine, Sapporo, Japan
e-mail: idogawa@sapmed.ac.jp

T. Saito
Department of Obstetrics and Gynecology, Sapporo Medical University School of Medicine, Sapporo, Japan
e-mail: tsaito@sapmed.ac.jp

H. Nakase
Department of Gastroenterology and Hepatology, Sapporo Medical University School of Medicine, Sapporo, Japan
e-mail: hiro_nakase@sapmed.ac.jp

A. Sakurai
Division of Clinical Genomics, Department of Genomic and Preventive Medicine, Sapporo Medical University School of Medicine, Sapporo, Japan

Genome Medical Center, Carres Memorial Hospital, Sapporo, Japan
e-mail: sakurai.akihiro@sapmed.ac.jp

M. Arai et al. (eds.), *Practical Guide to Hereditary Breast and Ovarian Cancer IV*,
https://doi.org/10.1007/978-981-95-6580-1_24

this general population dataset with those observed in the cancer-based Japanese Organization of Hereditary Breast and Ovarian Cancer registry, we identified an intriguing relationship with the status of companion diagnostic test reimbursement under the Japanese national health insurance system. In this manuscript, we present a full account of findings, along with additional analyses including the subsequently released ToMMo-60KJPN dataset.

Keywords Hereditary breast and ovarian cancer · ToMMo-54KJPN · ToMMo-60KJPN · Japanese Organization of Hereditary Breast and Ovarian Cancer · Companion diagnostic

1 Introduction

This chapter is based partly on our presentation at the Annual Meeting of the Japanese Organization of Hereditary Breast and Ovarian Cancer (JOHBOC) 2024 as well as a previously published paper [1]. In that study, we analyzed the ToMMo-54KJPN dataset, which contains whole-genome allele frequencies of single-nucleotide variants and indels obtained from approximately 54,000 individuals in the general Japanese population in the Tohoku region, as reported by the Tohoku Medical Megabank Organization (ToMMo) [2]. Our objective was to investigate the prevalence of pathogenic *BRCA1/2* variants in the general Japanese population.

Inherited pathogenic variants in *BRCA1* and *BRCA2* are well known to confer elevated susceptibility to breast and ovarian cancers, collectively recognized as hereditary breast and ovarian cancer syndrome (HBOC) [3]. Therefore, understanding how common these pathogenic variants are in the general population is a major public health concern. In Japan, analyses of patient cohorts and their relatives registered through JOHBOC have highlighted several possible founder mutations [4, 5]. Yet global surveys indicate that these variants occur less frequently outside Japan, underscoring the importance of population-specific genomic studies within the country [6]. Therefore, it is essential to accumulate data from population-based studies unique to Japan. In the present study, we analyzed the 54KJPN dataset for *BRCA1/2* variants in order to elucidate the frequency of HBOC in the general Japanese population.

2 Methods and Variant Frequencies

To estimate the carrier frequencies of HBOC-associated variants, we extracted *BRCA1* and *BRCA2* sequence changes from the ToMMo-54KJPN dataset. Reference transcripts applied for annotation were NM_007294.4 for BRCA1 and NM_000059.4 for *BRCA2*. Within these genomic loci, we identified 7711 distinct BRCA1 variants and 6320 unique *BRCA2* variants. Annotation was performed using ANNOVAR software [7] with the ClinVar dataset (20,230,702, https://ftp.ncbi.nlm.nih.gov/pub/clinvar/vcf_GRCh38/), as previously described [8]. Among the variants, 37 in *BRCA1* and 55 in *BRCA2* are predicted to be pathogenic or likely pathogenic, according to the ClinVar criteria. Furthermore, all truncating variants that were unclassified in ClinVar were evaluated and classified as pathogenic, based on the ENIGMA classification criteria. Although we similarly evaluated several truncating variants that were classified as being of uncertain significance or conflicting in ClinVar, their classification did not change. Assuming that each variant occurs independently (given the very low maximum allele frequency of 3.96×10^{-4}) and that the probability of an individual carrying two or more variants is negligible, all allele counts for *BRCA1* and *BRCA2* were aggregated. The estimated carrier frequencies, based on pathogenic/likely pathogenic ClinVar variants, were 2.485×10^{-3} for *BRCA1*, 2.873×10^{-3} for *BRCA2*, and 5.350×10^{-3} for either *BRCA1* or *BRCA2*. When truncating the variants classified as pathogenic according to the ENIGMA criteria were also included, the frequencies increased to 2.577×10^{-3}, 3.204×10^{-3}, and 5.772×10^{-3}, respectively. Although the presentation at this annual meeting was based on the 54KJPN dataset, we also performed a new analysis, using the 60KJPN dataset—an update that includes genome data from approximately 6000 additional individuals (https://jmorp.megabank.tohoku.ac.jp/downloads/tommo-60kjpn-20240904-af_snvindelall). In the 60KJPN analysis, we identified 15 additional pathogenic variants in *BRCA1/2*, and the estimated carrier frequencies for all categories were higher compared with the 54KJPN data. Specifically, the frequencies rose to 2.735×10^{-3} (164/119,859.3) for BRCA1, 3.486×10^{-3} (209/119,815.0) for *BRCA2*, and 6.211×10^{-3} for carriers of pathogenic variants in either *BRCA1* or *BRCA2*, including those classified according to the ENIGMA criteria.

3 Results and Discussion

A distinct pattern emerges when comparing 54KJPN data from the JOHBOC registry, which focuses on *BRCA*-tested cancer cases and pedigree analysis [4, 5]. The most common *BRCA1* pathogenic variant in 54KJPN, *BRCA1*:c.188T>A (p.Leu63*), is also the most frequently reported in the JOHBOC registry [4]. The third most common variant, *BRCA1*:c.2800C>T (p.Q934*), is the second most frequent in the JOHBOC registry. However, *BRCA1*:c.5096G>A (p.R1699Q), which ranks second in pathogenic *BRCA1* variants in 54KJPN, is not listed as a founder variant in the JOHBOC registry (Fig. 1). This is likely due to the "intermediate risk" associated with this variant. Indeed, several studies have shown that the risk of breast and ovarian cancer for individuals carrying the *BRCA1*:c.5096G>A (p.R1699Q) variant is lower than that for variants involving the same amino acid (p.R1699W) or truncating variants [9, 10]. In general, population-based studies play

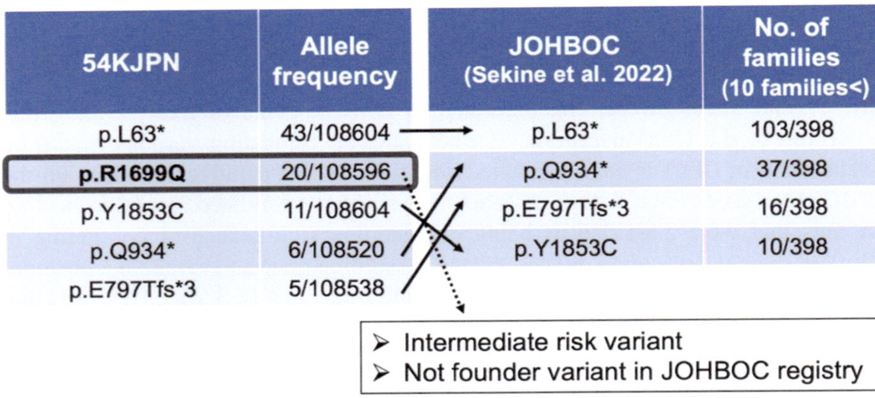

Fig. 1 Comparison to *BRCA1* variants in the JOHBOC registry: intermediate risk variant

a crucial role in identifying potential cancer risk groups that may be difficult to detect through cancer pedigree-based analysis.

Regarding *BRCA2* variants, the most common variant in 54KJPN, *BRCA2*:c.6952C>T (p.R2318*), is also the most frequent in the JOHBOC registry. However, it is worth noting that this variant did not seem to be a founder variant in the JOHBOC registry until 2018 and was found only in three pedigrees [5]. The reason for this significant change in ranking is likely due to the fact that BRACAnalysisCDx® and MyChoice CDx® companion diagnostic tests for ovarian cancer started to be covered by the Japanese national health insurance system in 2019 and 2021 (Fig. 2). These tests are now performed for almost all advanced ovarian cancer cases in order to determine eligibility for PARP inhibitor therapy, which has led to the rapid accumulation of *BRCA1/2* variant information related to ovarian cancer in the JOHBOC registry. However, BRACAnalysis® had been covered by insurance since 2018 for unresectable or recurrent breast cancer prior to ovarian cancer. This has led to temporal gaps in the clinical background of individuals undergoing testing. Pathogenic *BRCA1/2* variants have been categorized based on location, which is associated with increased risk of breast cancer (breast cancer cluster region) or ovarian cancer (ovarian cancer cluster region) [11], and *BRCA2*:c.6952C>T (p.R2318*) falls under the ovarian cancer cluster region category. Therefore, the accumulation of variants with a predominant history of breast or ovarian cancer may lead to bias in the types of *BRCA1/2* variants detected. Many of the variants detected in ToMMo-54KJPN were not frequently observed in the JOHBOC registry. As mentioned above, there might also be some intermediate-risk variants, suggesting that each cancer risk associated with detected variants might be heterogeneous. The accumulation of ongoing variant data and the follow-up of carriers with variants specific to the Japanese population might lead to the proposal of variant-specific surveillance and intervention strategies in the future.

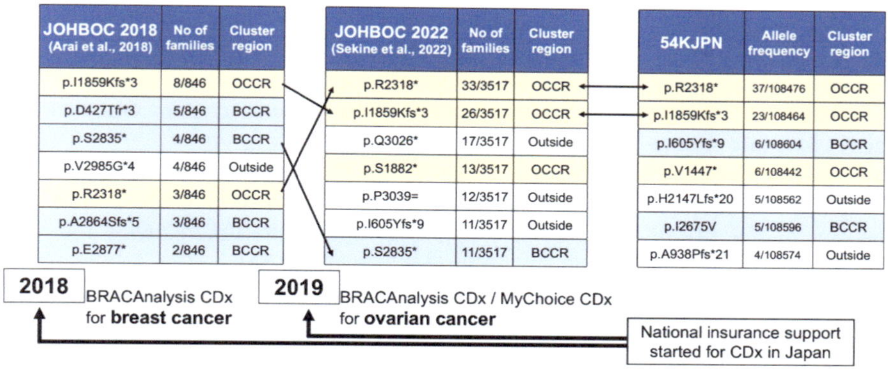

Fig. 2 Comparison to *BRCA2* variants in the JOHBOC registry: ovarian cancer cluster region/ breast cancer cluster region

It has been reported that approximately 10–20% of HBOC cancer patients who underwent germline testing harbor variants of uncertain significance (VUS) [12].

In ToMMo-54KJPN, variants classified in ClinVar as being of uncertain significance or conflicting interpretations of pathogenicity show allele frequencies of 36.8% in *BRCA1* and 8.4% in *BRCA2*, with the allele frequency being notably higher in *BRCA1*. This is due to the high allele frequency of the stop loss variant *BRCA1*:c.*873_*872delAA (rs59541324), which stands at 31.4%. Based on this frequency, it is thought that this variant is likely a non-pathogenic single-nucleotide polymorphism in the Japanese population, and it should be considered for reclassification to benign based on the results of this study. Generally, in the assessment and reclassification of VUS, in silico analyses predicting the impact of amino acid substitutions on protein folding play a crucial role [12, 13]. A novel in silico pathogenicity prediction algorithm for missense variants, called AlphaMissense, was recently introduced [14]. This algorithm combines the accurate in silico protein folding analysis algorithm AlphaFold2 based on deep learning with a protein language model. AlphaMissense resulted in the reclassification of some VUS in *BRCA1/2* genes as likely pathogenic (6.6%, 25/381 variants), although the majority were classified as likely benign (87.9%, 315/381 variants). It was suggested that many VUS are likely to be reclassified as likely benign through further observation and evaluation [15]. Therefore, the ability of the AlphaMissense algorithm to classify missense variants at a certain level of accuracy is expected to be highly valuable for future clinical management. More recently, a groundbreaking approach for reassessing VUS has been demonstrated for *BRCA2* variants. Studies by Sahu et al. [16] and Huang et al. [17] focused on the *BRCA2* DNA-binding domain, a VUS-enriched region essential for homologous recombination. Using saturation genome editing in mouse and human cells, those studies generated a comprehensive functional map of DNA-binding domain variants. Cross-referencing with the 60KJPN dataset revealed that most ClinVar-listed VUS in this region were classified as likely benign or benign, with only a few rated as likely pathogenic in one study, and none consistently classified as pathogenic. These findings underscore the value of saturation genome editing in clarifying the pathogenicity of VUS. This approach is expected to enable the elucidation of VUS and unclassified variants in other domains and genes in future studies.

Two large case-control studies in Japan, led by Momozawa and colleagues using Biobank Japan data, identified multiple founder variants, several of which were also present in the 54KJPN dataset [18, 19]. One variant, BRCA2:c.5645C>A, was absent from 54KJPN, likely due to differences in regional distribution. For example, BRCA1:c.188T>A and BRCA2:c.1813delA are more common in the Tohoku region, whereas BRCA2:c.5576_5579del is more frequent in the Kinki region [19]. Although Japan is an island nation without a land connection to the continent, regional variations in variant distribution may exist. Similar variations in the prevalence and characteristics of pathogenic variants across states have been reported in the United States [20, 21]. A limitation of the present study is that 54KJPN is derived solely from the Tohoku region and does not include clinical information, preventing pathogenicity assessments for noncoding variants.

4 Conclusion

Our findings clarify the prevalence and characteristics of *BRCA1/2* pathogenic variants in the Japanese population, reveal regional and clinical practice-driven differences, and underscore the potential of new technologies to resolve VUS. Continuous accumulation of nationwide data will be critical for precision cancer prevention and personalized risk management in HBOC.

Conflict of Interest There are no conflicts of interest to declare.

References

1. Idogawa M, Mariya T, Tanaka Y, Saito T, Nakase H, Tokino T, et al. The frequency and pathogenicity of BRCA1 and BRCA2 variants in the general Japanese population. J Hum Genet. 2024. https://doi.org/10.1038/s10038-024-01233-w.
2. Tadaka S, Hishinuma E, Komaki S, Motoike IN, Kawashima J, Saigusa D, et al. jMorp updates in 2020: large enhancement of multi-omics data resources on the general Japanese population. Nucleic Acids Res. 2021;49(D1):D536–D44. https://doi.org/10.1093/nar/gkaa1034.
3. Hu C, Hart SN, Gnanaolivu R, Huang H, Lee KY, Na J, et al. A population-based study of genes previously implicated in breast cancer. N Engl J Med. 2021;384(5):440–51. https://doi.org/10.1056/NEJMoa2005936.

4. Sekine M, Enomoto T, Arai M, Yokoyama S, Nomura H, Nishino K, et al. Correlation between the risk of ovarian cancer and BRCA recurrent pathogenic variants in Japan. J Hum Genet. 2022. https://doi.org/10.1038/s10038-021-01002-z.
5. Arai M, Yokoyama S, Watanabe C, Yoshida R, Kita M, Okawa M, et al. Genetic and clinical characteristics in Japanese hereditary breast and ovarian cancer: first report after establishment of HBOC registration system in Japan. J Hum Genet. 2018;63(4):447–57. https://doi.org/10.1038/s10038-017-0355-1.
6. Rebbeck TR, Friebel TM, Friedman E, Hamann U, Huo D, Kwong A, et al. Mutational spectrum in a worldwide study of 29,700 families with BRCA1 or BRCA2 mutations. Hum Mutat. 2018;39(5):593–620. https://doi.org/10.1002/humu.23406.
7. Wang K, Li M, Hakonarson H. ANNOVAR: functional annotation of genetic variants from high-throughput sequencing data. Nucleic Acids Res. 2010;38(16):e164. https://doi.org/10.1093/nar/gkq603.
8. Idogawa M, Hida T, Tanaka T, Ohira N, Tange S, Sasaki Y, et al. Renal angiomyolipoma (AML) harboring a missense mutation of TSC2 with copy-neutral loss of heterozygosity (CN-LOH). Cancer Biol Ther. 2020;21(4):315–9. https://doi.org/10.1080/15384047.2019.1702406.
9. Moghadasi S, Meeks HD, Vreeswijk MP, Janssen LA, Borg A, Ehrencrona H, et al. The BRCA1 c. 5096G>A p.Arg1699Gln (R1699Q) intermediate risk variant: breast and ovarian cancer risk estimation and recommendations for clinical management from the ENIGMA consortium. J Med Genet. 2018;55(1):15–20. https://doi.org/10.1136/jmedgenet-2017-104560.
10. Spurdle AB, Whiley PJ, Thompson B, Feng B, Healey S, Brown MA, et al. BRCA1 R1699Q variant displaying ambiguous functional abrogation confers intermediate breast and ovarian cancer risk. J Med Genet. 2012;49(8):525–32. https://doi.org/10.1136/jmedgenet-2012-101037.
11. Rebbeck TR, Mitra N, Wan F, Sinilnikova OM, Healey S, McGuffog L, et al. Association of type and location of BRCA1 and BRCA2 mutations with risk of breast and ovarian cancer. JAMA. 2015;313(13):1347–61. https://doi.org/10.1001/jama.2014.5985.
12. Fanale D, Pivetti A, Cancelliere D, Spera A, Bono M, Fiorino A, et al. BRCA1/2 variants of unknown significance in hereditary breast and ovarian cancer (HBOC) syndrome: looking for the hidden meaning. Crit Rev Oncol Hematol. 2022;172:103626. https://doi.org/10.1016/j.critrevonc.2022.103626.
13. Spurdle AB, Healey S, Devereau A, Hogervorst FB, Monteiro AN, Nathanson KL, et al. ENIGMA—evidence-based network for the interpretation of germline mutant alleles: an international initiative to evaluate risk and clinical significance associated with sequence variation in BRCA1 and BRCA2 genes. Hum Mutat. 2012;33(1):2–7. https://doi.org/10.1002/humu.21628.
14. Cheng J, Novati G, Pan J, Bycroft C, Zemgulyte A, Applebaum T, et al. Accurate proteome-wide missense variant effect prediction with AlphaMissense. Science. 2023;381(6664):eadg7492. https://doi.org/10.1126/science.adg7492.
15. Macklin S, Durand N, Atwal P, Hines S. Observed frequency and challenges of variant reclassification in a hereditary cancer clinic. Genet Med. 2018;20(3):346–50. https://doi.org/10.1038/gim.2017.207.
16. Sahu S, Galloux M, Southon E, Caylor D, Sullivan T, Arnaudi M, et al. Saturation genome editing-based clinical classification of BRCA2 variants. Nature. 2025. https://doi.org/10.1038/s41586-024-08349-1.
17. Huang H, Hu C, Na J, Hart SN, Gnanaolivu RD, Abozaid M, et al. Functional evaluation and clinical classification of BRCA2 variants. Nature. 2025. https://doi.org/10.1038/s41586-024-08388-8.
18. Momozawa Y, Iwasaki Y, Parsons MT, Kamatani Y, Takahashi A, Tamura C, et al. Germline pathogenic variants of 11 breast cancer genes in 7,051 Japanese patients and 11,241 controls. Nat Commun. 2018;9(1):4083. https://doi.org/10.1038/s41467-018-06581-8.

19. Momozawa Y, Sasai R, Usui Y, Shiraishi K, Iwasaki Y, Taniyama Y, et al. Expansion of cancer risk profile for BRCA1 and BRCA2 pathogenic variants. JAMA Oncol. 2022. https://doi.org/10.1001/jamaoncol.2022.0476.
20. O'Brien TD, Potter AB, Driscoll CC, Goh G, Letaw JH, McCabe S, et al. Population screening shows risk of inherited cancer and familial hypercholesterolemia in Oregon. Am J Hum Genet. 2023. https://doi.org/10.1016/j.ajhg.2023.06.014.
21. Grzymski JJ, Elhanan G, Morales Rosado JA, Smith E, Schlauch KA, Read R, et al. Population genetic screening efficiently identifies carriers of autosomal dominant diseases. Nat Med. 2020;26(8):1235–9. https://doi.org/10.1038/s41591-020-0982-5.

JOHBOC Registration

JOHBOC Registration, Registration Data of JOHBOC 2023

Takanori Ishida, Arisa Ueki, Narumi Harada-Shoji, Yoshiaki Akama, and Seigo Nakamura

Abstract In 2020, *BRCA1/2* genetic testing became covered by insurance in Japan for breast and ovarian cancer patients suspected of having hereditary breast and ovarian cancer (HBOC). At the same time, risk-reducing surgery also became available under insurance, leading to growing interest and expectations in genetic medicine. The Japanese Organization of Hereditary Breast and Ovarian Cancer (JOHBOC) operates a registry of HBOC patients and their families. The purpose of building the HBOC database is to clarify the genetic characteristics of Japanese individuals and to establish standard treatment practices. Participation is being encouraged from medical facilities throughout Japan.

This chapter summarizes the 2023 data. A total of 161 facilities nationwide took part in the registry project. The number of enrolled *BRCA1/2* pathogenic variant carriers was 4345. In addition, 451 patients underwent risk-reducing mastectomy (RRM), and 846 patients underwent risk-reducing salpingo-oophorectomy (RRSO). Since April 2020, surveillance, RRM, and RRSO for HBOC patients with a history

T. Ishida (✉)
Tohoku Kosai Hospital and Department of Breast and Endocrine Surgical Oncology, Tohoku University Graduate School of Medicine, Sendai, Miyagi, Japan
e-mail: takanori.ishida.a7@tohoku.ac.jp

A. Ueki
Department of Clinical Genetics, The Cancer Institute Hospital of Japanese Foundation for Cancer Research, Tokyo, Japan
e-mail: arisa.ueki@jfcr.or.jp

N. Harada-Shoji
Department of Breast and Endocrine Surgical Oncology, Tohoku University Graduate School of Medicine, Sendai, Miyagi, Japan
e-mail: narumi.harada.a3@tohoku.ac.jp

Y. Akama
Department of Clinical Genetics, Tochigi Cancer Center, Tochigi, Japan
e-mail: yoshiaka@tochigi-cc.jp

S. Nakamura
Department of Breast Surgical Oncology, Showa University School of Medicine, Tokyo, Japan

M. Arai et al. (eds.), *Practical Guide to Hereditary Breast and Ovarian Cancer IV*,
https://doi.org/10.1007/978-981-95-6580-1_25

of breast or ovarian cancer have been covered by insurance in Japan. Three years have passed since then, and the current state of HBOC care in Japan has gradually become clearer. However, HBOC care is still not covered by insurance for unaffected *BRCA1/2* pathogenic variant carriers. Nearly 500 such unaffected carriers have already been enrolled in this registry. Developing a medical care system for these individuals is now considered an urgent priority.

Keywords *BRCA1/2* · HBOC · Database · JOHBOC registry

1 Current Status of Japanese Genetic Medicine

It has become clear that approximately 5–10% of cancers are associated with a genetic predisposition. Among these, the most well-known are the *BRCA1/2* genes, which are implicated in multiple cancers, including breast and ovarian cancer. Furthermore, research on *BRCA1/2* has advanced, revealing their involvement in other cancers such as pancreatic, prostate, gastric, and biliary tract cancers.

In Japan, as of April 2020, patients diagnosed with breast or ovarian cancer that may be related to hereditary breast and ovarian cancer (HBOC) syndrome can receive *BRCA1/2* genetic testing covered by insurance, provided they meet certain criteria. At the same time, risk-reducing mastectomy (RRM), risk-reducing salpingo-oophorectomy (RRSO), and MRI surveillance for HBOC patients with a history of breast or ovarian cancer are now partially reimbursed by insurance.

The inclusion of preventive surgeries for asymptomatic individuals under insurance coverage represents a significant step forward in the field of genetic medicine in Japan. However, for individuals with *BRCA1/2* mutations who have not yet developed cancer, these preventive procedures are still not covered by insurance, which remains a significant issue.

2 Latest Status of JOHBOC Registration

The HBOC Consortium was established in 2012 with the aim of improving and expanding the medical system for patients with HBOC or suspected HBOC, as well as their families, thereby contributing to better medical care and preventive medicine across the country. Its philosophy and registered data were transferred to the Japanese Organization of Hereditary Breast and Ovarian Cancer (JOHBOC) in 2016.

One of the main initiatives of JOHBOC is the creation of a national registry for patients and families affected by hereditary breast and ovarian cancer. By compiling and tracking HBOC cases across Japan, the registry aims to clarify the clinical and genetic characteristics of HBOC—such as the features of *BRCA1/2* pathogenic mutations and the cancer incidence rates among mutation carriers.

In addition, by accumulating data on individuals with *BRCA1/2* pathogenic mutations through genetic testing, the project seeks to promote appropriate screening, diagnosis, and treatment strategies for patients and their families, with the ultimate goal of reducing mortality from breast, ovarian, and related cancers.

To achieve this, the JOHBOC registry project aims to establish a comprehensive database of hereditary breast and ovarian cancer, recruit medical institutions nationwide, and use the collected data to improve clinical guidelines and standardize care by reflecting the genetic and clinical characteristics of the Japanese population. Participating institutions must be capable of providing appropriate genetic counseling and testing for eligible patients. Based on the study protocol, information from patients and their families who have provided written informed consent using the designated information sheet and consent form will be registered.

3 JOHBOC Registration Details and Update Status

To support the long-term accumulation of cancer-related information and follow-up data, the registration data for all cases is updated annually, and a list of registered cases for each fiscal year is compiled at the end of August. Previously, *BRCA1/2* genetic test results and clinical information for patients and their relatives who underwent testing at participating medical centers were entered into the database. Since the 2022 registration cycle, the project has targeted patients and families who have undergone *BRCA1/2* genetic testing and been found to carry either a deleterious or suspected deleterious mutation, or a variant of unknown significance (VUS). For a detailed history of the registration project, please refer to the previous report [1–4].

Registrants are categorized into four groups:

1. Individuals who underwent *BRCA1/2* genetic testing at a participating facility
2. Individuals who were tested elsewhere but received treatment or follow-up at a participating facility
3. Blood relatives registered based on a proband's information
4. Others

If a participant is found to have been registered at another facility, and with their consent, the facilities will coordinate to minimize duplicate registration. In the following section, we present an overview of the nationwide registration data compiled as of September 2023.

4 Summary of JOHBOC Registration Data for 2023: Number of Registrations

Currently, 161 facilities are participating in this registry project, and a total of 4345 *BRCA1/2* pathogenic variant carriers who have attended these facilities have been registered (*BRCA1*: 2051; *BRCA2*: 2276; *BRCA1&2*: 18). In addition, 803

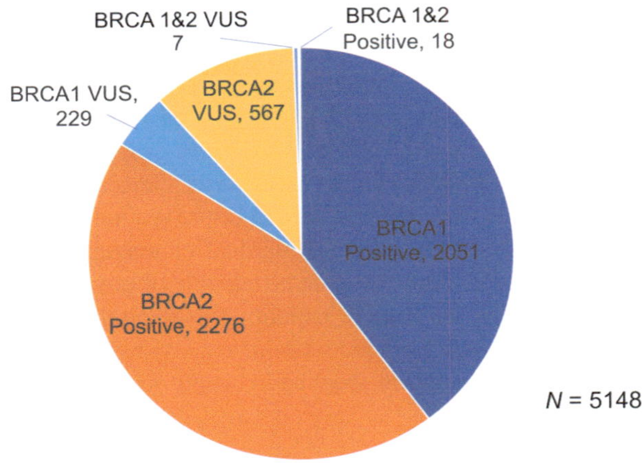

Fig. 1 Data collection study: pathogenic mutation & VUS

individuals with a variant of uncertain significance (VUS) in *BRCA1/2* have been enrolled (*BRCA1*: 229; *BRCA2*: 567; *BRCA1&2*: 7) (Fig. 1).

5 Summary of JOHBOC Registration Data for 2023: Registered Variants

A total of 380 distinct pathogenic variants of the *BRCA1* gene were registered (Table 1). The most frequently reported variant was c.188T>A (p.Leu63*), identified in 406 patients. This was followed by c.2800C>T (p.Gln934*), reported in 140 patients, and c.2389_2390del (p.Glu797Thrfs*3), reported in 52 patients (Table 2).

Similarly, 386 distinct pathogenic variants of the *BRCA2* gene were registered (Table 1). The most common was c.6952C>T (p.Arg2318*), found in 226 patients, followed by c.5576_5579del (p.Ile1859Lysfs*3) in 199 patients, and c.9076C>T (p.Gln3026*) in 101 patients (Table 3).

For variants of VUS, 129 distinct variants were registered for the *BRCA1* gene and 234 for the *BRCA2* gene (Table 1).

Table 1 Registered variants: 2023

BRCA1		
Interpretation	Variants	No. of cases
1	380	1611
2	34	155
3	129	247
Total	553	2013
BRCA2		
Interpretation	Variants	No. of cases
1	386	1990
2	10	75
3	234	580
Total	630	2645

1. Deleterious
2. Suspected Deleterious
3. VUS

Table 2 *BRCA1* pathogenic variant with the highest number of registrations

Exon	HGVS cDNA	HGVS protein	No. of cases
5	c.188T>A	p.Leu63*	406
11	c.2800C>T	p.Gln934*	140
11	c.2389_2390del	p.Glu797Thrfs*3	52
24	c.5558A>G	p.Tyr1853Cys	35
3	c.131_132del	p.Cys44*	31
11	c.3442del	p.Glu1148Argfs*7	26
11	c.2075_2076del	p.His692Argfs*19	24
16	c.4964C>T	p.Ser1655Phe	24
19	c.5154G>T	p.Trp1718Cys	24
20	c.5278-1G>A		20

Table 3 *BRCA2* pathogenic variant with the highest number of registrations

Exon	HGVS cDNA	HGVS protein	No. of cases
13	c.6952C>T	p.Arg2318*	226
11	c.5576_5579del	p.Ile1859Lysfs*3	199
23	c.9076C>T	p.Gln3026*	101
10	c.1813del	p.Ile605Tyrfs*9	88
11	c.5645C>A	p.Ser1882*	77
20	c.8504C>A	p.Ser2835*	73
18	c.8023A>G	p.Ile2675Val	63
23	c.9117G>A	p.Pro3039=	53
10	c.1278del	p.Asp427Thrfs*3	49
11	c.6405_6409del	p.Asn2135Lysfs*3	40

6 Ipsilateral Breast Cancers in *BRCA1/2* Pathogenic Variant Carriers

Among *BRCA1/2* pathogenic variant carriers who developed breast cancer, 714 women who underwent breast-conserving surgery were available for follow-up after genetic testing. Of these, ipsilateral breast cancer was observed in 8 *BRCA1* carriers, 10 *BRCA2* carriers, and 5 carriers of both *BRCA1* and *BRCA2* after genetic testing (Table 4).

The follow-up periods after genetic testing range (mean, median) were as follows: for *BRCA1*, 0.1–20.4 years (mean 2.3, median 0.5); for *BRCA2*, 0.1–19.0 years (mean 2.1, median 0.4); and for *BRCA1 & 2*, 0.1–1.4 years (mean 0.8, median 0.6).

The annual incidence rates of ipsilateral breast cancer were 1.0%/year for *BRCA1* carriers, 1.3%/year for *BRCA2* carriers, and 0%/year for carriers of both *BRCA1* and *BRCA2*.

Table 4 Ipsilateral breast cancers in *BRCA1/2* pathogenic variant carriers

	BRCA1&2	BRCA1	BRCA2	VUS
Breast-conserving surgery cases	5 cases	343 cases	366 cases	214 cases
Ipsilateral breast cancer after the genetic testing	0 case	8 cases	10 cases	4 cases
Observation period after the genetic testing (mean, median)	0.1 ~ 1.4 years (0.8, 0.6)	0.1 ~ 20.4 years (2.3, 0.5)	0.1 ~ 19.0 years (2.1, 0.4)	0.1 ~ 14.6 years (1.4, 0.4)
Incident rate (%/year)	0/4.1 0%/year	8/801.8 1.0%/year	10/775.1 1.3%/year	4/302.3 1.3%/year
Background				
Age at first onset of breast cancer (in years) (average)	38 ~ 55 (46.6)	23 ~ 80 (41.9)	19 ~ 81 (45.4)	25 ~ 91 (46.9)

Table 5 Contralateral breast cancers in *BRCA1/2* pathogenic variant carriers

	BRCA1&2	BRCA1	BRCA2	VUS
Unilateral breast cancer incidence (traceable cases)	10 cases	939 cases	1213 cases	568 cases
Contralateral breast cancer after genetic testing	1 case	32 cases	34 cases	2 cases
Observation period after the genetic testing (mean, median)	0.1 ~ 14.1 years (3.1, 1.1)	0.1 ~ 20.0 years (2.0, 0.8)	0.1 ~ 23.4 years (1.9, 0.5)	0.1 ~ 22.2 years (1.2, 0.5)
Incident rate (%/year)	1/30.8 3.2%/year	32/1856.6 1.7%/year	34/2301.0 1.5%/year	2/698.5 0.29%/year
Background				
Age at first onset of breast cancer (in years) (average)	32 ~ 78 years (47.6 years)	21 ~ 85 years (43.4 years)	19 ~ 83 years (44.6 years)	23 ~ 91 years (46.8 years)

7 Contralateral Breast Cancers in *BRCA1/2* Pathogenic Variant Carriers

A total of 2162 women with unilateral breast cancer and *BRCA1/2* pathogenic variants were available for follow-up after genetic testing. Of these, 67 developed contralateral breast cancer after genetic testing (Table 5).

The follow-up periods after genetic testing range (mean, median) were as follows: for *BRCA1*, 0.1–20.0 years (mean 2.0, median 0.8); for *BRCA2*, 0.1–23.4 years (mean 1.9, median 0.5); and for *BRCA1* & *BRCA2*, 0.1–14.1 years (mean 3.1, median 1.1).

The annual incidence rates of contralateral breast cancer were 1.7%/year for *BRCA1* carriers, 1.5%/year for *BRCA2* carriers, and 3.2%/year for carriers of both *BRCA1* and *BRCA2*.

8 Risk-Reducing Surgery

A total of 451 *BRCA1/2* pathogenic variant carriers underwent risk-reducing mastectomy (RRM) (*BRCA1*: 249; *BRCA2*: 200; *BRCA1* & *2*: 2). Of these, 416 (91.4%) underwent contralateral RRM and 39 (8.6%) underwent bilateral RRM. The mean age at RRM was 55.0 years. Occult breast cancer was detected in 8.0% of the participants (*BRCA1*: 3.5%; *BRCA2*: 4.5%).

In addition, 846 *BRCA1/2* pathogenic variant carriers underwent risk-reducing salpingo-oophorectomy (RRSO) (*BRCA1*: 435; *BRCA2*: 406; *BRCA1* & *2*: 5). The mean age at RRSO was 49.8 years. Occult ovarian cancer was detected in 1.5% of the participants who underwent RRSO (*BRCA1*: 0.9%; *BRCA2*: 0.6%).

Table 6 Prostate cancer and pancreatic cancer in *BRCA1/2* pathogenic variant carriers

	BRCA1&2	BRCA1	BRCA2
No. of male pathogenic variant carriers	0	65	152
Prostate cancer incidence (cases)	0	8	49
Incident rate (%)	0	12.3%	32.2%
	BRCA1&2	BRCA1	BRCA2
No. of pathogenic variant carriers	18	2051	2276
Pancreatic cancer incidence (cases)	0	18	63
Incident rate (%)	0	0.88%	2.8%

9 Prostate Cancer and Pancreatic Cancer in *BRCA1/2* Pathogenic Variant Carriers

A total of 217 male *BRCA1/2* pathogenic variant carriers were registered. Of these, 8 of 65 *BRCA1*-positive cases and 49 of 152 *BRCA2*-positive cases developed prostate cancer after genetic testing. The incidence rates were *BRCA1*: 12.3% and *BRCA2*: 32.2% (Table 6).

In addition, 4345 *BRCA1/2* pathogenic variant carriers were registered for pancreatic cancer analysis. Of these, 18 of 2051 *BRCA1*-positive cases and 63 of 2276 *BRCA2*-positive cases developed pancreatic cancer after genetic testing. No cases of pancreatic cancer were observed among 18 carriers of both *BRCA1* and *BRCA2* pathogenic variants. The incidence rates were *BRCA1*: 0.88% and *BRCA2*: 2.8% (Table 6).

From 2024, a new data entry system will be implemented to allow for more detailed registration of prostate cancer and pancreatic cancer cases.

10 Follow-Up Data of *BRCA1/2* Pathogenic Variant Carriers

A total of 491 unaffected *BRCA1/2* pathogenic variant carriers were registered. Of these, 310 could be followed after genetic testing, yielding a follow-up rate of 63.1%. In addition, 272 *BRCA1/2* pathogenic variant carriers who developed cancer after genetic testing were registered, with a follow-up rate of 80.1%. The follow-up rates in both groups remain insufficient for a comprehensive analysis of the genetic characteristics of the Japanese population, highlighting the need for continued accumulation of follow-up data.

11 Research Issues Using Data from the JOHBOC Registry

This registry project aims to provide new knowledge to medical professionals through publications and presentations at academic conferences based on the database. Clinical research proposals are solicited annually from participating facilities that meet specific criteria, such as registering follow-up data. The research theme and lead presenter are determined through discussions by the Registry Committee and the Academic Committee, with approximately two to three proposals selected each year.

The selected proposals are presented at an academic conference hosted by JOHBOC and subsequently published as papers. However, due to delays in the analysis and manuscript preparation of studies adopted before 2022, no new research proposals were accepted in 2023.

12 Future Outlook

The improved data entry system for this registry project has facilitated the long-term accumulation of follow-up data on registrants, gradually clarifying the current status of *BRCA1/2* pathogenic variant carriers in the Japanese population. Furthermore, starting in fiscal year 2024, a new data entry system will be implemented to enable more detailed registration of information regarding prostate and pancreatic cancers. It is expected that data on these cancers will be accumulated alongside existing data on breast and ovarian cancers.

Moving forward, it will be necessary to effectively utilize this data and advocate for insurance coverage of appropriate surveillance and risk-reducing surgery for unaffected *BRCA1/2* pathogenic variant carriers. To accomplish this, continued accumulation of follow-up data is essential, and the importance of this must be clearly communicated to participating institutions.

Acknowledgements JOHBOC Registration Committee: [Committee]: Arisa Ueki (Cancer Institute Hospital), Yoshinori Akama (Tochigi Cancer Center), Hiroki Den (Showa University), Narumi Harada (Tohoku University), Takeo Kosaka (Keio University), Hiraku Kumamaru (Tokyo University), Chigusa Morizane (National Cancer Center Hospital), Masato Ozaka (Cancer Institute Hospital), Ayumi Shikama (Tsukuba University), Kanae Taruno (Showa University). [Secretariat of JOHBOC]: Eriko Shimamoto (Showa University), Mieko Takeuchi (Showa University). Participating 161 institutions that entered their data with our 2023 registry: Yamagata Prefectural Central Hospital, Shiroyama Hospital, Nihonkai General Hospital, Saitama Medical University International Medical Center, Fukushima Medical University, Japanese Red Cross Aichi Medical Center Nagoya Daini Hospital, Yamaguchi University, Tohoku University Hospital, Kanagawa Cancer Center, Tosei General Hospital, Gunma Prefectural Cancer Center, Hoshi General Hospital, Kansai Rosai Hospital, Seirei Hamamatsu General Hospital, Yokohama City University, Nagasaki University, National Hospital Organization Kyoto Medical Center, Japanese Red Cross Saitama Hospital, Japanese Red Cross Yamaguchi Hospital, Saitama Medical Center, National Hospital Organization Osaka National Hospital, Osaka University, Yamanashi Prefectural Central Hospital, Aichi Cancer Center Hospital, St. Luke's Hospital, Shikoku Medical Center for Children and Adults, Japanese Red Cross Medical Center, Nippon Medical School Musashi Kosugi Hospital, St. Marianna University School of Medicine, University of Miyazaki Hospital, The Jikei University, Shikoku Cancer Center, Hiroshima Prefectural Hospital, Hokkaido University, Kitano Hospital, Keio University, Japanese Red Cross Ishinomaki Hospital, JA Hiroshima General Hospital, Kokura Medical Center, Saku Medical Center, Showa Medical University Hospital, Tottori University, Kitasato University, Shizuoka Cancer Center, Tokuyama Central Hospital, University of Tsukuba,

Japanese Red Cross Nagoya Daiichi Hospital, Ibaraki Prefectural Hospital, Nagoya University, Okayama University, Fujita Medical University, Chiba University, Sapporo Medical University, Saiseikai Hyogoken Hospital, Shonan Memorial Hospital, Iwate Medical University, Kawasaki Medical School, Saitama Cancer Center, Juntendo University, Fukui University, Nagoya City University, Shizuoka General Hospital, Shinshu University, Nara Medical University, Kitakyushu Municipal Medical Center, Tokyo Medical Center, Sagara Hospital Breast Center, Hiroshima University, Gifu University, Kochi Medical Center, Cancer Institute Hospital, JCHO Saitama Medical Center, Asahikawa Medical University, Kyoto University, Osaka International Cancer Institute, Ishikawa Prefectural Central Hospital, Hyogo Medical University, Okazaki City Hospital, Kochi University, Tawara IVF Clinic, Niigata University, Ehime University, Jisenkai Aizawa Hospital, Shizuoka municipal Hospital, Toranomon Hospital, Japan Community Healthcare Organization Sagamino Hospital, Kansai Medical University, Tokushima University Hospital, Kanazawa University, Nara Prefecture General Medical Center, Ogaki Municipal Hospital, Oikawa Hospital, Kagawa University Hospital, Tokyo Metropolitan Komagome Hospital, Nippon Medical School, Hokkaido Cancer Center, Mie University Hospital, Yamagata University Hospital, Toyota Memorial Hospital, National Center for Global Health and Medicine, Toyama University Hospital, Hyogo Prefectural Amagasaki General Medical Center, Matsushita Memorial Hospital, Kagawa Prefectural Central Hospital, Hamamatsu University School of Medicine, University Hospital, Hyogo Cancer Center, Medical Journal of Japanese Red Cross Society Wakayama Medical Center, Osaka Metropolitan University Hospital, Kagoshima University Hospital, Hamamatsu Medical Center, Fujisawa City Hospital, Tokyo Saiseikai Central Hospital, Kindai University Hospital, Yamaguchi Rosai Hospital, Fukui Prefectural Hospital, Sekishindo Hospital, JA Onomichi General Hospital, Aichi Medical University Hospital, Yokohama City University Medical Center, Kato Breast Surgery Clinic, Kansai Electric Power Hospital, Kyoto Miniren Chuo Hospital, Kanazawa Medical University Hospital, National Hospital Organization Kyushu Medical Center, Sapporo Tokushukai Hospital, University Of Yamanashi Hospital, Nishiwaki Municipal Hospital, Akita University Hospital, Showa University Koto Toyosu Hospital, Matsue City Hospital, Matsue Red Cross Hospital, Suwa Red Cross Hospital, Aomori Prefectural Central Hospital, Osaka Police Hospital, Osaka Red Cross Hospital, Osaka General Hospital of West Japan Railway Company, Osaki Citizen Hospital, Kyoto City Hospital, Tottori Prefectural Central Hospital, Toyama Prefectural Central Hospital, Fukuoka University Hospital, Fukuoka Wajiro Hospital, Toyohashi Municipal Hospital, Nagoya Ekisaikai Hospital, Niigata Prefectural Central Hospital, Nagano Red Cross Hospital, Konan Medical Center, Gifu Prefectural General Medical Center, Kyoto Prefectural University of Medicine Hospital, Shimane University Hospital, Tokyo Women's Medical University, Toho University Ohashi Medical Center, Shikokai Medical Corporation Mitsubishi Kyoto Hospital, Kobe City Medical Center General Hospital, Tachikawa Hospital, Federation of National Public Service Personnel Mutual Aid Associations, Nagahama Red Cross Hospital, Takatsuki General Hospital, Aijinkai Healthcare Corporation, The University of Tokyo Hospital, Shimane Prefectural Central Hospital, Akita Red Cross Hospital, Tsuchiura Kyodo General Hospital.

References

1. Arai M, Yokoyama S, Watanabe C, et al. Genetic and clinical characteristics in Japanese hereditary breast and ovarian cancer: first report after establishment of HBOC registration system in Japan. J Hum Genet. 2018;63(4):447–57.
2. Arai M, The Registration Committee of the Japanese Organization of Hereditary Breast and Ovarian Cancer (JOHBOC). Hereditary Breast and Ovarian Cancer. Hereditary Breast and Ovarian Cancer (HBOC) database in Japan. In: Nakamura S, Aoki D, Miki Y, editors.

Hereditary breast and ovarian cancer molecular mechanism and clinical practice. Springer Singapore; 2021. p. 243–57.
3. Inuzuka M, Arai M, Nakamura S. Registration data of Japanese Organization of Hereditary Breast and Ovarian Cancer till 2020. In: Aoki D, Nakamura S, Miki Y, editors. Practical guide to hereditary breast and ovarian cancer annual meeting of the Japanese Organization of Hereditary Breast and Ovarian Cancer 2021. Springer Singapore; 2023. p. 145–54.
4. Inuzuka M, Ishida T, Nakamura S. Updates to the registration data of the Japanese Organization of Hereditary Breast and Ovarian Cancer: summary for 2022. In: Ohta T, Iwata H, Suzuki N, Nakamura S, editors. Practical guide to Hereditary Breast and Ovarian Cancer Annual Meeting of the Japanese Organization of Hereditary Breast and Ovarian Cancer 2022. Springer Singapore; 2024. p. 119–26.

MIX
Papier aus verantwortungsvollen Quellen
Paper from responsible sources
FSC® C105338

If you have any concerns about our products,
you can contact us on
ProductSafety@springernature.com

In case Publisher is established outside the EU,
the EU authorized representative is:
Springer Nature Customer Service Center GmbH
Europaplatz 3, 69115 Heidelberg, Germany

Printed by Libri Plureos GmbH
in Hamburg, Germany